PHYSICAL THERAPY MA

NEW PATIENT
ACCELERATOR METHOD

HOW I SCALED A FOUR LOCATION, $1,000,000 +
CASH PAY PHYSICAL THERAPY CLINIC
– IN A PLACE WHERE HEALTH CARE IS FREE
(...AND, IN ONE OF THE POOREST PARTS OF THE
COUNTRY)

PAUL GOUGH

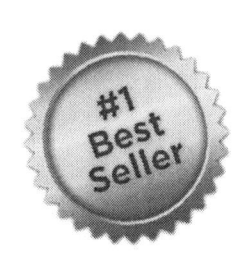

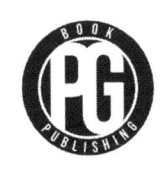

Paul Gough Publishing

Copyright © 2018 Paul Gough. All rights reserved.

This publication is licensed to the individual reader only. Duplication or distribution by any means, including email, disk, photocopy, and recording, to a person other than the original purchaser, is a violation of international copyright law.

Publisher: Paul Gough, 25 Raby Road, Hartlepool, UK, TS24 8AS

While they have made every effort to verify the information here, neither the author nor the publisher assumes any responsibility for errors in, omissions from or a different interpretation of the subject matter. This information may be subject to varying laws and practices in different areas, states, and countries. The reader assumes all responsibility for the use of the information.

The author and publisher shall in no event be held liable to any party for any damages arising directly or indirectly from any use of this material. Every effort has been made to accurately represent this product and its potential and there is no guarantee that you will earn any money using these techniques.

ISBN-10: 978-1721139088

ISBN-13: 1721139087

DEDICATION

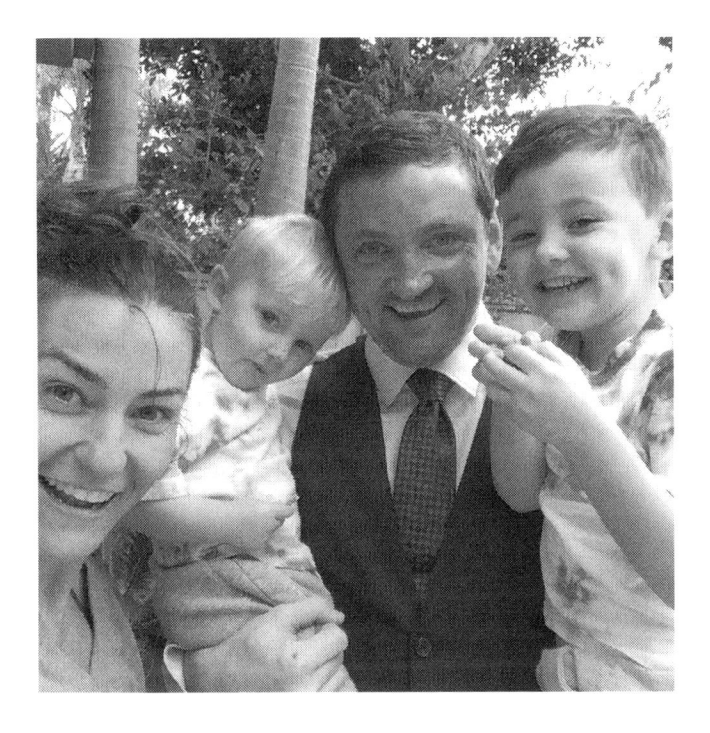

To Natalie, Harry and Tobias – it is my wish that this book impacts your life just as much as the people who read it.

I love you all
xxx

To my clients – all over the world - thank you for the trust you have placed in me and for giving me the opportunity to help you.

It means the world to me.

BEFORE YOU READ THE BOOK DO THIS FIRST...

Just to say thanks for reading this book **I would like to give you the sample Facebook, newspaper and postcard ads, training videos, system blueprints, and worksheets** that are mentioned within the book – absolutely FREE!

Go to: **www.paulgough.com/resource**
to download it now.

Here's What You Will Receive:

- **My No.1 performing Facebook and newspaper ads** - just copy and paste into your clinic's next marketing campaign

- **Your first Free Report/Lead Magnet** – start attracting your perfect patients instantly with this done for you free report

- **Complete resources from the book**, including all the links, system blueprints and even more bonuses that I have not mentioned here

It's All Here:

www.paulgough.com/resource

YOU'LL NEED THIS AS YOU READ THE BOOK...

Go to: **www.paulgough.com/resource** now and download your FREE bonus Marketing Tool Kit PDF - it contains many of the ads that I mention in the book...

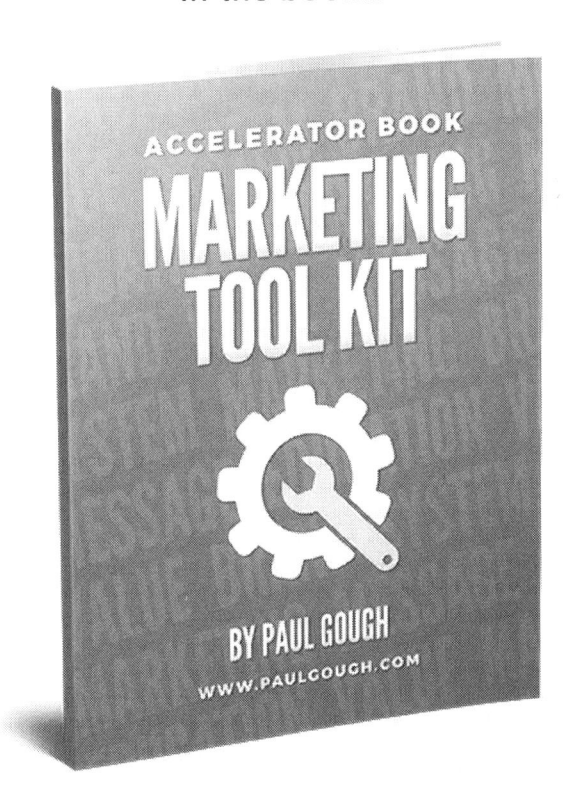

To get the best out of this book download the resource PDF now before you start reading:
www.paulgough.com/resource

PRAISE FOR PAUL GOUGH AND THE ACCELERATOR METHOD MARKETING SYSTEM (FROM PHYSICAL THERAPISTS ALL OVER THE WORLD)

....

"Before taking Paul's Accelerator program I wasn't even making $4000 in a month as a solo-cash PT – 15 months on from taking the class and I've since made $19,700 in cash, in ONE WEEK, using his marketing methods and my business continues to grow, month on month."
Kevin Vandi, Competitive Edge PT, San Jose, Ca

"If you want strategies to help reduce or eliminate your insurance headaches, Paul is the person to show you how – he has concrete ideas to implement rather than strictly theory like so many other PT marketing people. We have been able to drop almost all of the insurance companies thanks to what Paul showed us on Accelerator."
Kim Gladfelter PhysioFit Physical Therapy, Los Altos, Ca

"I've worked with Paul for over 3 years now. He is refreshingly honest, straightforward and easy to talk to and I love his no-nonsense approach to direct marketing. You'll find with Paul that he is up front about what to expect, and more importantly, he is honest enough to tell you what NOT to expect. There are no false promises with Paul. I've recommend him to many other PT owners who have been equally impressed with their results."
Dean Volk, Volk PT, Concord, NC

"Before meeting Paul I was stressed, unhappy, underpaid and underappreciated at my Mill Like PT Clinic – Accelerator gave me the confidence to quit my job and just 3 months on I'm already making more in a month working for myself than I ever was at my job. Thank you Paul!"
Kevin Mao, Balance and Restoration, San Francisco, Ca

"Paul's approach is completely different, it's ethical and customer driven. I love the fact that everything he teaches you on Accelerator is what he is doing at his own clinic – and that the strategies actually WORK!"
Judith Mcloughlin, Body-Dynamic, Brighton, UK

"I've only implemented one third of what Paul taught me to do - and I already feel the difference. Paul style marketing definitely WORKS!"
Carrie Jose, CJ Physical Therapy and Pilates, Portsmouth, NH

"Paul's energy and enthusiasm for business is infectious. Learning from him has made me a better person and a better business owner and taking Accelerator was what really reignited my fire for growing my company".
Wendy McCloud, WDC Physiotherapy, Essex, UK

"I started a cash-based practice and it wasn't long before I was "stuck" with no calls and no patients – Paul style marketing has been my "cure!"
Christine Walker, Christine Walker Physical Therapy, Harrisburg, NC

"When I first spoke to Paul I was in a small room in a rented facility seeing just one or two patients per week – I took Accelerator and within 14 months I went from charging $150 per session to $225, had 60 visits + per week on schedule, I hired my first full time staff PT and had moved into my own premises. Whatever Paul tells me to do – I just do it! That's because every time I speak to Paul - I make more money."
Jake Berman, Berman Physical Therapy, Naples FL

"Paul is the "Marketing MASTER" of our profession and over the last 3 years I've had the pleasure of learning from him and all of the great work he has done at my practice. Most importantly, I have found a true friend who is as genuine and down to earth as anyone I know!"
Andrew Vertson, Intecore PT, CA

"Paul teaches you the stuff that isn't taught in school at all. His teaching has had a serious impact on all of the clinics in our franchise and across Quebec since working with him."
Alain Sheldeman, Action Sport Physiotherapy, Montreal, Canada

"Paul is a marketing genius. I learn something from him every time we speak. To be able to compete against FREE is amazing… the marketing tips, techniques and mind-set offered by Paul are absolute gold!!"
Dr. Jarod Carter, Cash PT, Austin TX

"We went from charging $175 per session – to charging $450 in cash using Paul's Accelerator marketing system, in less than 12 months!"
Oscar Andalon, Level4PT, Encinitas, CA

"Paul shows you how to market a successful business in today's healthcare economy. Accelerator has completely changed how I market my clinic. If you want to set up a system to market your practice, I don't think there is a better teacher out there."
Julietta Wenzel, Ocean Therapy Centre, Wilton Manners, FL

"Accelerator was fantastic! I don't normally get excited when I write reviews/give feedback but you deserve it – I resonate with your passion and preach your words to my staff regularly, which is great, because it means you are having a profound effect on my whole business. We are "pumping out" more visits than ever since we took your class and I've got the other partners in my business wanting to know what has changed – our marketing is what has changed!"
Nick Young, Benchmark Physiotherapy, Sydney, Australia

"I took Paul's Accelerator Program and it was hands down the best marketing training I have ever taken."
Aaron LeBauer, LeBauer Physical Therapy, Greensboro, NJ

"There's only one person I would ever trust with my marketing – and that is Paul Gough."
Jerry Durham, San Francisco Sport And Spine, CA

"I spent years chasing Doctors for referrals – I got more new patients within 3 weeks of taking Accelerator than I did in all that time chasing the Doctors."
Oliver Patalinghug, Restore PT, Rochester Hills, MI

"Since taking Accelerator my monthly revenue has increased by 60%. I was seeing 7 patients a week and just 13 months on, I'm now at capacity and charging $100 more per visit and ready to make my first full time hire!"
Trupti Mehta, Manual Medicine PT, Washington D.C

"My revenue has doubled since taking Accelerator and because it is all about Systems I have a lot more time to work ON the business (not in the business), and to spend with my family!"
Nick Hunter, Preferred PT, Glendale, AZ

"Most PTs are now aware of the huge crowd of people that Paul teaches you to market to – Accelerator shows you how to address that opportunity."
Neil Sauer, Functional Advantage, Hemlock, MI

"Until Accelerator, I have literally never had a patient come to me that has not been from a referral from a Doctor or from doing a talk, in my entire career. This course changed all that and Paul's method has shown me how to acquire new patients from multiple different sources."
Justin Rabinowitz, Chiropractor, Strive2Move, Warren, NJ

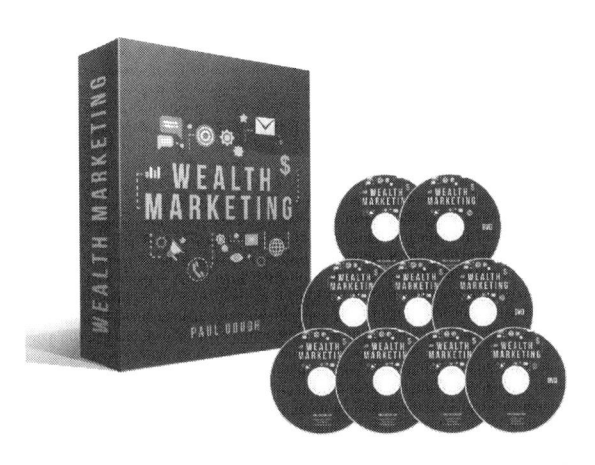

GET YOUR FREE WEALTH MARKETING GIFT FROM PAUL, NOW...

Go to: **www.paulgough.com/wealth-gift**
To get this instant access 9 DVD video program, NOW

Claim your $1,997.00 worth of cash patient generating, higher profit making, wealth marketing DVD program, absolutely FREE!

Including a FREE "Test-Drive" of Paul Gough's Cash Club Membership that sends to your clinic $10,000 worth of marketing ideas every 30 days.

**Claim your copy now, at
www.paulgough.com/wealth-gift**

CONTENTS

INTRODUCTION

Why Most Physical Therapy Clinic Marketing Fails - 1

CHAPTER 1

Could Everything You've Ever Been Told About Marketing Your Physical Therapy Clinic Be Wrong? - 9

CHAPTER 2

If This Can Work in a Free, Socialist Healthcare System, Can it Work For You? - 31

CHAPTER 3

How to Increase Your Profit 10x Using Lead Generation Marketing - 45

CHAPTER 4

How to Attract Patients Happy to Pay Cash - 61

CHAPTER 5

Finding the Fortune Already in Your Clinic - 85

CHAPTER 6

3 Steps to Grow Your Practice Profits
Using Marketing That Actually Works - 103

CHAPTER 7

Where to Find an Endless Supply of Your Perfect Patients - 119

CHAPTER 8

How to Get Paid Faster –
Turn Inquiries Into High Paying Patients, Fast - 145

CHAPTER 9

The Cash Value Maximization System - 163

CHAPTER 10

Getting Into the $100K Club - 179

INTRODUCTION

WHY MOST PHYSICAL THERAPY CLINIC MARKETING FAILS

If you are like most people you learned the same things I did at school about marketing a physical therapy practice: **nothing**.

Sadly, you're allowed to start a physical therapy practice thinking that the only way to get new patients is to bake cookies or provide luncheons for the doctors and hope that yours taste better than everyone else's. If they don't like the cookies, the next thing to do is send them a newsletter and hope they read it. If that doesn't work, you're told to keep sending them more newsletters in the hope you get past the gate-keeper (receptionist), and if you can't do that, up the offering with a weekly luncheon for the entire staff at the doctor's office.

And if you don't get the referrals after that – try it all again. But this time around, you do it with a different doctor, in a different part of town, in the hope that this one is hungry when you call, or that he or she likes reading newsletters with information that is nothing more than a blatant sales pitch for your clinic.

When will this madness stop?

The belief that you need to market to doctors, or remain trapped inside of the insurance system, is built into the culture of our profession. We are taught to worship the doctors and accept peanuts from insurance companies who care more about their profits than your patients' care – as if there is no other choice.

Building relationships with doctors is idealized, and having more of them refer to you is how you are led to believe this is the only way to grow a private practice.

But what if there was another way? What if it could be easier than having to relentlessly suck up to the doctors, bake cakes and cookies, and accept chickenfeed from low-paying insurance companies who pay barely enough to keep the doors open – never mind take home a profit?

What if there was a way where patients could choose you on merit - because you offer the most value and are able to provide the outcome they hope for, and, in return, they'd be happy to pay you a fee that YOU set – one that allows you to make a profit that doesn't just cover your college debt?

WHY IS THIS IMPORTANT TO YOU NOW?

In my experience, almost everything I've been taught about marketing and growing a physical therapy clinic is either wrong, out-of-date, or even if it does "work", it leads to a debt and stress ridden practice owner with hardly any life or energy left when they arrive home at the end of the day.

After quitting a high-profile job as a physical therapist working in professional soccer, I started my practice in my mid-20s and I was quickly sucked into the insurance rat-race, and not long after I found myself working longer hours with less take home pay than I was earning in my previous job.

It took me nearly seven years to realize that everything I'd ever been told about how to market and grow my practice was wrong – and because of that I was destined to end up like most owners who are broke, stressed, and unhappy, only ever seeing their kids after they have gone to bed, and all this in the name of growing a business that will one day "pay out".

It cost me tens of thousands of dollars and countless hours in wasted advertising efforts to learn that almost everything that everyone was telling me to do when it came to marketing my practice could never possibly work.

And what's worse, it took me two years of being **stuck**, feeling burned out, and suffering a suspected heart attack (at the age of just 31) to force me to learn how market my practice correctly.

In the pages of this book I am going to share with you everything I've learned about marketing and running a successful business – and how I was able to walk away from all of the hassle and heartache that a typical business owner feels as though they have to live with, by giving you the exact system I use.

THE TYPICAL JOURNEY OF A TYPICAL PHYSICAL THERAPY CLINIC OWNER...

I am pleased that you picked this book up when you did...

If you are a cash based clinic owner, a lack of marketing know-how has likely put you in a situation where you've started a clinic but you have no predictable or reliable method for acquiring new patients. Some weeks you get calls, but most weeks you don't. The doctors won't even consider you so you are working hard, knocking on doors asking for referrals from other fitness business owners, and you're likely working your social media network channels to advertise to all of your followers that you are "open for business."

And it works. But only to a point.

There's no sustainable growth or feeling of control, and you certainly do not feel confident enough to scale, hire, or move to a better premises. And as for raising your prices – you are too fearful to do that just in case you lose the next one or anger the ones you've got.

If that is **you**, you are already well and truly STUCK and it is vital you read this book.

And if you are a traditional insurance based clinic owner, not knowing how to market directly to the public has most likely left you trapped inside of the system; you have **decreasing profit margins**, doctors are getting harder to reach, and you're forced to work harder for less take home pay than most of the staff you employ. You are doing the lunches thing, you're doing the newsletters thing, and during all this you are watching and waiting for the letter to come from the next insurance company giving you good news: your reimbursements are being reviewed (lowered), and that there's nothing you can do about it.

If that is you, I suspect you are asking yourself daily "what is the point of it all?" Possibly even questioning whether or not you should just go back to working for someone else (so that they can deal with the worry and hassle that you currently have), wondering why you don't just throw in the towel, so that you can walk out the door at 5pm each night with a guaranteed salary (like your staff do). Am I warm?

If that is you, you will love this book and the strategy that I am sharing with you. I'll show you how to stop focusing on getting more patients, and start focusing on more PROFIT instead.

WHAT HAPPENS TO CLINICS THAT DO NOT HAVE A MARKETING SYSTEM

Take a look at the image on the next page – it may resonate with you…

FIG.1

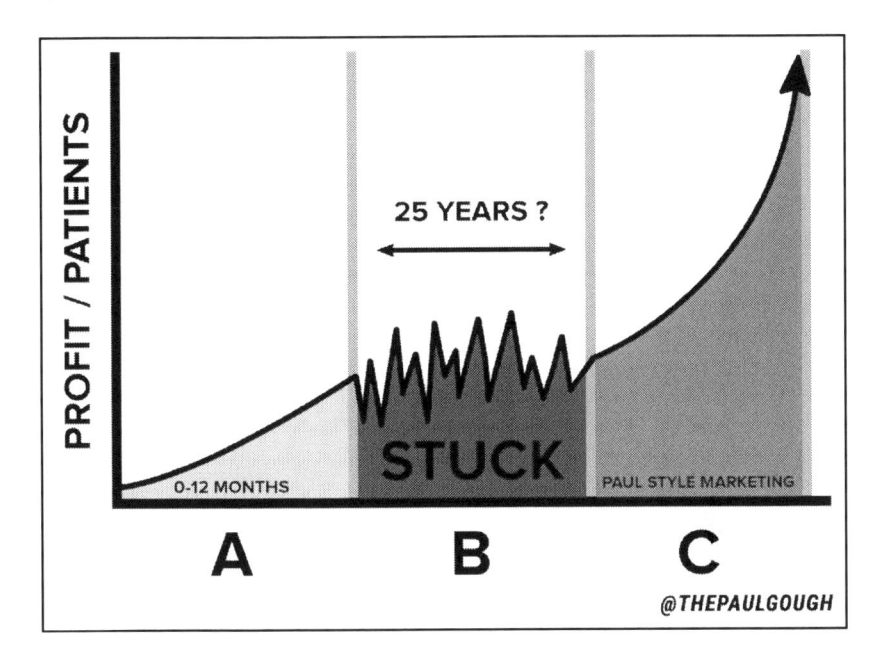

Figure: A graph with PROFIT / PATIENTS on the y-axis, divided into three zones A, B, and C. Zone A (0-12 MONTHS) shows gradual growth. Zone B shows erratic "STUCK" pattern labeled "25 YEARS?". Zone C (PAUL STYLE MARKETING) shows steep upward growth. Tagged @THEPAULGOUGH.

It is an accurate representation of how physical therapy businesses start - and then get "stuck" - <u>due to the owner's lack of marketing skill or know-how</u>.

In the first 0-12 months (ZONE A) it is all about "hard work" and "hustle" – the "go-to" strategy for most fledgling clinic owners. That strategy gets you started, but it also gets you stuck. Knocking on doors, speaking to gym owners, doing your workshops, and building up your social media presence is a great way to start. However, all of that without a real marketing system to bring in new leads predictably and reliably, causes that same clinic owner to get "stuck" in ZONE B; this is where most, if not all owners remain for the rest of their career.

It is a case of "boom or bust", or "feast or famine": a few busy weeks treating patients followed by lots of slow weeks when you didn't have time to hustle or knock on doors. And so it goes on for decades. Revenue is unpredictable in this state and there is little, if any profit. The slow weeks break you more than the good weeks make you, and at the end of the year you wonder why, despite working so hard, there's hardly any noticeable difference in your take home salary.

Can you relate?

It is no way to run a business, and yet the mantra of more "hard work" and more "hustle" has become the default mode of the profession. The solution is not to "keep working harder", nor is it to go bed even later, or get up any earlier than you are right now.

Here's a novel idea: how about you stop trying to do more of what isn't working and just **change the strategy?**

THIS IS A MARKETING BOOK - NOT A RECIPE BOOK

I want to make it clear from the outset so that there can be no confusion; this is a marketing book - **not a cookbook**.

That means there will be no recipes for baking cookies or ways to serve luncheons to the doctors. Those guys make enough money to cover their own lunches, and besides, they've never fed me or my family – why should I feed them or theirs?

I mean this respectfully when I say that the profession has caused its own downfall by relying too heavily, and for too long, on a single referral source. And now that the tide has gone, or is fast going out, many clinic owners are being caught out; they've been swimming naked for too long and now they're being exposed.

What you will find in this book is a completely new marketing strategy to get you "unstuck" (if you are already there) and avoid getting stuck (if you think you are heading that way). And if you feel like you are trapped inside the system with no way out, this is a proven method of making more profit in your business and still getting home by 5 o'clock each night.

GOOD MEDICINE RARELY TASTES NICE

Everything you are about to read in this book is fact – **not theory**.

I have made this work in my own clinic first, and I've since shown 11,531 (at the time of printing) physical therapists, from **all across America and in 14 other countries, how to do it as well.**

This strategy is precisely how I have grown my own business (The Paul Gough Physio Rooms) from scratch to $1m + in revenue, in a county with free socialist medicine. I have risked my own time and money to learn all of what you are about to discover, and my clinic continues to use the same strategy that you are about to learn to grow its profits year on year – without me having to be there every day.

This entire book is based upon what I have done (and what I continue to do) to take a clinic that was stuck, relying upon low paying third party referrals, and always waiting to get paid off insurance companies, to one that has made a healthy **six figure profit** year after year without working in it. These days I decide when I go home for dinner, and having this system I am about to share with you is the primary reason I am able to be present with, and spend quality time with my family and two beautiful boys any time I like. And just as fun, it has allowed me to tell most of the crappy insurance companies who stopped me from making a profit to go and shove their ridiculously low reimbursements where the sun doesn't shine.

I think the exact words I used in the letters I wrote to end my relationship with them were "go to hell".

Every single thing I will teach you is something I have paid the price to learn and then made work at my practice. I am sharing with you <u>results</u> (that work today), not my opinion (or what worked 5 or 10 years ago.)

To my knowledge I am one of the <u>**world's first**</u> physical therapy clinic owners who has been able to successfully **SCALE A CASH**

BASED BUSINESS past one location, and in the pages of this book I will share with you precisely how I did it.

I've since helped many others to do the same and I am sure you can do it too.

It is highly likely that throughout this book I am going to say things that you will not like or will not agree with. And that is great. When it happens, please remember that although you may not like the taste of the medicine the doctor prescribes, you know full well that it is **good for you** in the long run.

I know that at times you will be tempted to say to yourself things like, "I don't think that will work for me", or tell yourself "but my town is different". By predicting that in advance I am challenging you to **read this book with an open mind,** and instead of telling yourself "this won't work for me", ask yourself, "how could I make this work for me?" If/when you find you are "doubting" any of what you read, remember that thousands of others just like you are **DOING IT** and **CHANGING THEIR LIVES!**

Although my accent may be different to yours, how you build a successful business is no different no matter where you live or what type of clinic you run. In-fact, if you DO think it is somehow different where you are, or that your clinic is somehow unique and your challenges are different, I put it to you that is why you might not be as successful as you would like to be… For your own sake, give this system a fair trial. After all, what alternatives have you got?...

It is either this Accelerator system or it's back to the recipe books for the cookies, back to the lunches for the doctors, or back to accepting reimbursements that barely cover costs.

Enjoy the book.

1

COULD EVERYTHING YOU'VE EVER BEEN TOLD ABOUT MARKETING YOUR PHYSICAL THERAPY CLINIC BE WRONG?

Most physical therapy clinic marketing is doomed to fail. It is not because the ad isn't big enough, it is not because it doesn't look nice enough, and it is not because the logo isn't in the right place. It's simply because the ad campaign lacks a clear understanding of "who" it is that they are trying to target. There's no what I call "clear target market", and without a clear identification of your target market your marketing will not work.

Now I know what you are thinking, "but Paul, I am trying to attract <u>anyone</u> who is in pain. Everybody and anybody who is in any pain could be one of my patients!" If you are anything like me when I first started trying to market my clinic, you are probably thinking that all you have to do to create a successful marketing campaign is get in front of anyone who is in pain with an ad that says something like, "I am a qualified, friendly and experienced physical therapist and I provide quality customer service. I can ease your pain fast – call today for an appointment!"

If so, this is the **No.1 biggest mistake you can ever make with your marketing,** and if you have ever tried marketing to the public and it didn't work, it was most likely that you spent more time talking about yourself than what you can do or who you can do it for. Advertising credentials, experiences, and that you're a "friendly and professional clinic" is the go-to marketing strategy for most clinic owners trying to get going with their direct to public marketing.

There's no attempt to talk to a specific, pre-identified pocket of people (a "target market"), and therefore the marketing message nearly always fails to show how they can solve the target market's unique and specific problems.

IT'S NOT ABOUT YOU – IT'S ABOUT THEM

Here's the thing: marketing is not about advertising how you "pride yourself on great service", or even about showcasing how many years you've been in business. It is not about telling people how qualified you are and <u>it is not even about asking people to book an appointment.</u>

It is much simpler than all of that. If all of that sounds strange (particularly the not booking an appointment part) then congratulations – you've already learned a lesson that most business owners never get to learn in their whole life and one that might just save you a lot of heartache and wasted marketing dollars.

I wish I had learned it earlier… I wasted tens of thousands of dollars and countless hours running unsuccessful marketing campaigns to finally learn that marketing is not about me – it is about them. A "rookie" marketing mistake is to think that marketing is about announcing to the world that you exist. It is the "if you build it, then they will come" mentality, only this time it is "if I announce it, they will come".

But they don't.

THE 3 FUNDAMENTAL RULES OF DIRECT MARKETING SUCCESS

Successful marketing for physical therapy practices follows 3 fundamental rules:

1. **You have to be clear on who your perfect patient is**
2. **You have to say the right things to your perfect patient**

3. You have to reach your perfect patient in the places where they are

To make it simple, here's how they all fit and work together:

FIG.2

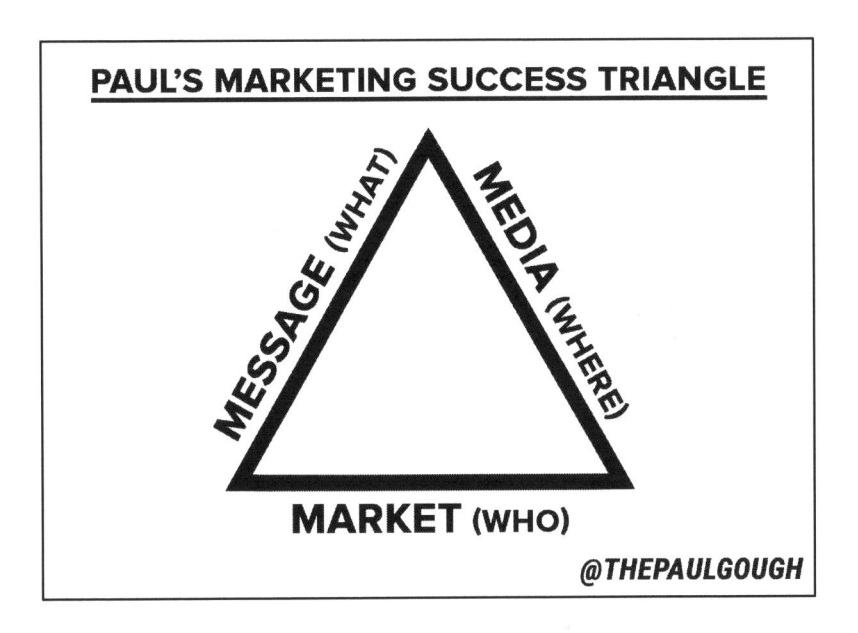

PAUL'S MARKETING SUCCESS TRIANGLE

MESSAGE (WHAT)
MEDIA (WHERE)
MARKET (WHO)

@THEPAULGOUGH

The usual scenario in most clinics is to decide to run an ad out of necessity because the patient volume is looking low, or even worse, the local newspaper called and offered a discount on a spot in the health feature that weekend. Neither is ideal, and the reason why is because there's zero thought ever going into the strategy about **"who"** is being targeted, what **"offer"** will be made to them, or even if the **"media"** used is where the ideal target market (perfect patient) is going to be looking.

These are the 3 fundamental rules of direct marketing success and they are all being ignored in favor of a time sensitive need to fill up the schedule or a looming deadline.

The only thought is to make the ad look aesthetically appealing and obsess over the color, the position of the logo, the font size and type, and have a designer dress it up with some attractive images.

Let me show you an example of what I mean - and YES, this was one of my own **from the early days** when I was dabbling with my clinics marketing:

FIG.3

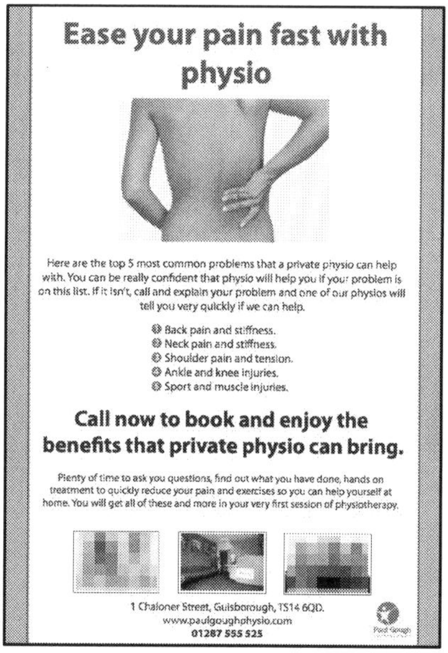

> **Ease your pain fast with physio**
>
> Here are the top 5 most common problems that a private physio can help with. You can be really confident that physio will help you if your problem is on this list. If it isn't, call and explain your problem and one of our physios will tell you very quickly if we can help.
>
> - Back pain and stiffness.
> - Neck pain and stiffness.
> - Shoulder pain and tension.
> - Ankle and knee injuries.
> - Sport and muscle injuries.
>
> **Call now to book and enjoy the benefits that private physio can bring.**
>
> Plenty of time to ask you questions, find out what you have done, hands on treatment to quickly reduce your pain and exercises so you can help yourself at home. You will get all of these and more in your very first session of physiotherapy.
>
> 1 Chaloner Street, Guisborough, TS14 6QD.
> www.paulgoughphysio.com
> 01287 555 525

Having spent all that time designing it the ad now "looks" perfect, the clinic owner is certain it represents his or her "brand identity" perfectly, and he can be sure that when everyone sees the ad, the phone is going to ring off the hook.

Except it doesn't.

Then what happens next is this: the business owner, still reeling at the loss of the $500 it cost to run the ad, (and the disappointment of being rejected, and heartache of being overlooked), decides that the solution to the marketing issue must be to change the color, change the font, and perhaps make the ad a little bigger, as maybe the reason that no one called was that no one noticed it?

So the new, bigger, more visually appealing ad runs. The business owner is even more convinced that they've got the "look and feel" of the ad right, and he is beyond certain that this time the phone will ring off the hook.

Except it doesn't.

There's rarely an attempt at ad number 3. Instead, what happens next is to blame the marketing itself (to cover up the business owners inept marketing skill) and a retreat back into the comfort zone of the old fashioned methods of marketing (to doctors or past patients) that didn't work back then, but now, because the direct marketing isn't working either, appears to be the only option.

"MARKETING DOESN'T WORK IN MY TOWN"

Here's the worst bit about a lack of early marketing success: the business owner, still scared from the loss and disappointment of the failed marketing campaign, now concludes that "marketing doesn't work in my town" or that "marketing doesn't work for physical therapy clinics". He is convinced that the only way to grow is to do what everyone else does - market to doctors or wait for referrals from past patients.

With that way of thinking the business owner is now sentenced to a lifetime of perpetual struggle doing what everyone else does, and getting what everyone else gets – a practice struggling to make a profit.

I appreciate that some people are addicted to that struggle – but I assure you, it does not have to be that way. And, if any of that sounds familiar then you are not alone, as this is pretty much the same mistake that I made, and it is how my first two years trying to market my clinic directly to the public looked.

Thankfully though I discovered that marketing does work in my town and it does work for physical therapy clinics – I just needed to change what I was doing and how I was doing it. I needed to change the strategy.

I needed to accept that I couldn't help anybody and everybody in pain and I needed to get clear on **"who"** it was I wanted to talk to (my target market). Once I knew that, it made it much easier to change the message in my ad.

I realized that words are powerful, and much like going on a first date, if I talked more about me (than her), I wouldn't get a second one. The same is true with marketing. The ads have to talk more about them than you and you have to give them a reason to get in touch with you that is more exciting and less risky than the "call now to book an appointment" phrase that was the ruin of nearly every ad I ever ran.

MARKETING MISTAKE #1: MARKETING TO THE WRONG GROUP OF PEOPLE

So, rule number 1 of marketing is that you have to get clear on **"who"** it is that you want to market to. This is called your **"target market"**, or as I will often refer to throughout this book, your **"perfect patient"**.

It took me a while to realize that there's only ever a very small pocket of people who are actively considering your services at any one time – that is despite significantly many more people needing it. The difference between "actively looking" and "needing" is huge. The number of people actively looking is so small that it makes marketing success almost impossible.

So the WHO that you should be targeting with your marketing is defined as a pocket of people who are suffering with a problem that you can solve, but who are, and this is the phrase to remember, **"not ready to book just yet"**.

The only thing that currently stands in the way of them booking that appointment with you is information about what you do and how their questions will be answered. Your new marketing strategy is about focusing on this group of people and providing them with the information they need to make an appointment with you. And the good news is, there's literally thousands of them in your town right now, and they are currently being overlooked by all your competition.

"WHY NO ONE RESPONDS TO TRADITIONAL ADS"

I remember the first time I heard this I was a little taken back. It took a while for this concept to sink in: there was a massive group of people out there who I could help but who simply were not ready to book an appointment. So, if this is the first time you are hearing anything like this, let me explain it a little more. No matter where you live or what type of business you run, **there are really only three different types of people** seeing your marketing ads:

Group 1 - Those not interested in your service and who don't need it (i.e. they have no pain or movement loss so they don't require your services or skills)

Group 2 - Those who need your services (i.e. because they have pain or movement loss), but who currently do not know you can help them, that you exist, or how to access your services

Group 3 - Those who need what you do and are actively looking and ready to book an appointment with you now (i.e. the ones everyone in business want more of)

JUST 3% READY TO BOOK NOW

Here's what is interesting: of the three types of people I just described, the group that most clinics focus on is the third group - the ones who need you and are ready to book an appointment now.

It makes sense that you would focus on them, right? After all they are the ones who are actively looking for a physical therapist and who want to hand over money in exchange for your service.

However, it is the wrong group to focus on, here's why - statistically, there is only ever around 3% of the population ready and confident enough to buy any product or service at any given time. That means if you sell TV's, only 3% of the market place, on any given day, are ready to buy. The other 97% walking into the store that day are just browsing. They are looking for information to start the buying process. It's the same with cars - right now, only 3% of people looking on websites or visiting car show rooms are in a position to buy a car today. The fact is most people buy a car after the third time looking.

Imagine how much more successful all of these companies would be if they took the approach that when a person walks into the show room it does not automatically mean they are customers – it means they are starting to make a decision. **Big difference.** The implications for how you would treat these people (in Group 2) are huge.

What does this mean for your practice? It means that any time you are creating a marketing campaign that says something like: "We're an affordable, friendly clinic - call today to book an appointment", you are talking to the third group of people – the smallest – which statistically gives you the least chance of being successful. Sure, they are the ones who are ready to say yes, but that group is so small that it is almost impossible to find them.

What is the best group? Group 2 – the ones who have a problem you can solve (i.e. back pain), but they just don't know enough to confidently say yes and call you… yet!

Statistically, there are around 30% of these people at any one time in any market place. That is 10x more potential patients for your business. How much more successful would you be if you had 10x the number of inquiries you are getting right now?

WHY THEY WILL NEVER BOOK IF ALL YOU EVER DO IS TALK ABOUT YOURSELF

To demonstrate this concept, I want to you to play along with me as I describe a likely scenario that is happening to both you and I every day. Picture yourself in your clinic; now, let's take a walk outside and stand at the front door. If your clinic is in a sports center or a medical facility, imagine that we are at the main entrance of the building. Look at all the people walking or driving past. For every 100 of them, I would bet that at least 30 have a problem that you know how to solve. It could be low-back or knee pain, pelvic floor dysfunction, a sports injury – tension headaches or migraine – whatever it is, I am sure that 30 of these people could and should be your patients.

The million dollar question is, why <u>aren't</u> they? The answer is they have no clue what you do.

They are not confident about walking in and asking for an appointment. They are thinking that tomorrow their pain will go away. They have been told to rest and take pills. They are thinking about calling a chiropractor or a massage therapist.

Whatever the problem is, they are your potential new patients, yet they are not coming to see you and no matter how big your "call today to book an appointment ad" is, they won't.

I have four clinics and two of them have a very visual frontage. There is high foot traffic and high visibility with hundreds of people walking and thousands of cars going past each day. It is not possible that of the hundreds of people who see my clinic each day, at least 30% don't have a problem I can solve. Yet very few actually call in to ask about making an appointment.

And this happens in-spite of a huge sign above the door saying "Physiotherapy Clinic", and many smaller signs in the huge glass windows talking about how we help things like back pain, knee pain, sports injuries, etc.

MARKETING MISTAKE #2: SAYING THE WRONG THINGS IN YOUR MARKETING

So what is really going on here – why don't they come in and see me? I am right there in front of them. They see me every day. I am right there – all they have to do is walk in and ask me to help. Well, I started to understand this more thanks to the help of a patient of mine called Christine.

This lady would walk past one of my clinics every day and eventually told me that she had walked past most days (truth be told, she had limped past most days) yet because she had been to see her doctor about her knee pain, and because that same doctor told her to "rest" and "just do some exercise when the pain goes", she thought "nothing could be done".

Those were her exact words. After all, if physical therapy was a viable option, then surely the doctor would have mentioned it?

ANOTHER LADY TOLD BY HER DOCTOR SHE "DIDN'T NEED PHYSICAL THERAPY"

She knew nothing of what physical therapists actually do, and it took her nearly two years to pluck up the courage to come into my clinic and ask the question about if we could help her or not.

Essentially, what happened was that her knee pain and frustration got so bad that she was willing to take the risk and pluck up the courage to call me. It was a last ditch attempt to solve the problem, which was born out of sheer frustration that two years of worrying about daily knee pain had caused. Not an ideal situation receive a patient – but it is a very common one when you stop to think about it.

Here's where this gets interesting: just imagine if the sign in the windows of my clinic had said something like this, "Have you been told by your doctor to just take pills and accept knee pain?"... What impact do you think that message would have had on Christine? Do you think she would have come to see me years earlier if I had wrote something like that in my clinic windows? (I think so too).

What changed here was the "marketing message". This is what you say in your ads about who you can help, and how you can help them. It is what dictates if people view you as an option (or not at all).

My ads were not working because the marketing message was non-existent. In fact it was not aimed at anyone, and it wasn't talking about solving a specific problem. I was trying to compete with everyone, for everyone, and it wasn't working.

So, what is the lesson to be learned here for your clinics marketing? It is that most clinics are failing at their marketing because there is no **"message to market match"**. The message to market match is achieved when you pre-identify a specific pocket of people you want to help and you say something that resonates with them so that they can come to their own conclusion that you are the right option they need.

When I look at the marketing being done by most clinics, in most cases I could sum it up like this: the wrong things are being said to the wrong people at the wrong time, and so a lack of response is inevitable.

In the example of Christine, "book an appointment now" would never have caused Christine to come and see me, no matter how big or attractive looking the ad was.

And that is a problem when you are trying to grow, because as you now know there are a lot more Christine's around than people who are actively looking to hire you today (remember, she is in Group 2).

NOT ONLY WAS I FOCUSING ON THE WRONG PERSON, I WAS FOCUSING ON THE WRONG PROBLEM!

Here's another story like that:

I have a patient called Mary. She is in her 50's, she loves to keep herself active and mobile, wants to avoid painkillers, and wants to maintain her independence as long as possible. She is the perfect patient for my practice. She's the type of patient that when she walks through the doors you wish you could find more of 'her'. She is so easy to work with, values what you do, and most importantly is happy to pay your fees.

One day I asked Mary for a video testimonial for my website. She agreed. I set up the camera after her final treatment session and I asked her a series of questions. It was only when I was watching the interview replay that it hit me why marketing was never going to work – not only was I focusing on the wrong person, **I was focusing on solving the wrong problem.**

I was trying to appeal to people with severe pain or movement dysfunctions, and that meant I was being overlooked by the people who I really wanted to work with.

"PAUL, I'M NOT IN ALL THAT MUCH PAIN"

So what did Mary say that day that had such a profound effect on my marketing? Well, when I asked her what her pain was like before she came to see me, here's what she said:

"Paul, I wasn't in that much pain. I was just frustrated with all of these 'niggly little injuries' that seem to be taking a toll on me. I am worried that I am going to have to slow down or miss out on family things. I found myself taking more and more painkillers, and I don't want to be spending my whole life taking them, so I decided to call you to see if you could help."

After listening back to what Mary had to say I realized why my clinic had "flat lined". Given that Mary is my perfect patient and I want to see more people like her, everything I was saying in my clinic's marketing message back then was actually repelling her (not attracting her).

I could have taken out the biggest newspaper ad in the Washington Post, or even a 60 second TV commercial during half time of the Super Bowl, but if I had spoken about how my service helps people in pain, or with motion loss, Mary would not have given the ad a second thought. After all, in her own words, the words of my most perfect patient, "she wasn't in all that much pain", she was just fed up and frustrated at her "niggly little injuries" which were slowing her down.

This is important for you to note, because the only thing that matters in marketing is how the customer sees what you are offering and how they see what they want. This perfect patient wasn't in all that much pain – she was being slowed down by lots of little problems all adding up. Big difference.

We might want them to have more function, increased ROM, and a VAS score of less than "2/10". The problem is, if all they want is to be able to play with their grandkids at the swing park this weekend, our grand vision for them is misaligned and leads to a negative outcome for both parties - the patient and clinic.

MARKETING MISTAKE #3: ASKING THEM TO DO THE WRONG THINGS

In both of these scenarios, no matter how experienced or how qualified I said I was, I wasn't getting the call if I focused my marketing on solving "pain" and asking people to "call" me, and yet this is how most clinics continue to market.

The group of people that gives me the most chance of increased ROI from my marketing is the group that don't really know enough about what I do to confidently say yes. They need me – there's just no trust there yet.

That means I need to change something else in my ad. If there's no trust there and there's a lack of understanding, you can't just use your ads to ask people to book appointments. That is asking people to take a huge leap of faith with you, and most people are very unlikely to ever want to do that.

Instead, you have to focus on building a relationship with the likes of Mary and Christine, and you have to use your marketing to talk about how you understand the challenges and struggles that they are living with. Make it easy for them to begin that relationship with you.

It is one thing having the "target market" reading and liking your compelling marketing message designed specifically for them – but, it is another to get them to respond to it. Importantly, what determines the response to the ad is something named the **"call to action",** or what is often termed, the "offer".

This "call to action" is the part of the ad where you ask the person (in the target market) who has resonated with what you said in your ad, (your marketing message), to do something that moves them closer to becoming a patient.

Offering to give them free "information" (like a "how to ease back pain in 7 simple steps" tips report) is by far the lowest risk offer you can make, and will increase your response rates tenfold. It is not asking them to commit to anything – only to take the first baby-steps to get in touch with you. You'll find that your response is inversely proportional to the level of "risk" involved in what you ask them to do in your ad.

Marketing mistake number 3 is to think that, just because you ask them to call you to book an appointment, they will. For all sorts of reasons like fear, doubt, or lack of confidence or trust, most wont. To get more calls from your ads, we have to make it very easy for them to take action. We do this by offering them something of perceived value that is of interest to them; something that helps them start solving their problem. What's more, we have to give them an incentive to call you (free from the risk of getting "sold to" or having to make a big commitment with you) so that more people feel more confident about making that decision.

'Information style reports' will do this better than anything else; there's more on how we do this later in the book. For now though I need you to understand that if you want to get more response from your marketing, <u>you have to stop asking for appointments</u> and start building bridges by offering information. When you do that you not only get a better response from your ads, but you also inherit far more compliant patients. It is win-win.

MARKETING MISTAKE NUMBER #4: THINKING YOU CAN PUT YOUR ADS ANYWHERE

Marketing mistake number 4 is to think that your ads can be successful anywhere.

They can't.

Now that you know "who" you want to target, and what you are going to say, the final part of the marketing triangle is to pick the media. For example the media could be newspapers, Facebook, or Google. You are asking yourself, "will my target market see the ad if I run it there?"

For example, would your 65-year-old perfect patient have more chance of seeing your ad in the newspaper or on Facebook? And, would the 25-year-old athlete who loves to do CrossFit see your ad in the newspaper or, much more likely on Instagram?

The answer is that either could work – but I know which one I am more likely to have success with simply by asking myself the question "does my target market use this media we are about to run this ad in or on"?

Tied with letting people tell you that you are competing with everybody for everybody who is in pain, the next worse thing you can do is think that you can put your ads anywhere. In theory you can. But in reality there's a high probability that doing it won't give you the response that you are looking for.

Given the option of theory or reality – I prefer reality all day long.

MARKETING MISTAKE NUMBER #5: NO LEAD GENERATION SYSTEM

You cannot grow any business without a system for predictable lead generation. A failure to have one is why so many clinics struggle and flat line. Sure, you might be able to "grow" your clinic on referrals from doctors (or third party payers) but my guess is that if you've gone down that route then you are possibly bigger, but are now operating with significantly less of a profit margin.

When you exist on referrals from doctors (or any third party) you are tirelessly trapped inside of "The System".

How do you know if you are trapped inside of the system? It's simple – you are at the mercy of other people when it comes to what you can charge and how much you can make. This is the real price you will pay for not having a lead generation system that produces your own supply of patients (happy to pay in cash). It is a business restricted by what it can charge, suffering with tighter profit margins year on year.

I know many insurance-based business that are growing bigger by the year – but they are also getting less and less profitable. As reimbursements go down, your costs are going up -as re-payments get less, the amount you have to pay out (on staff, rates, rent etc.,) is rising accordingly. That is inefficient growth with more work and less pay for the business owner, and there's only so long you can sustain it before the lights eventually go out.

It is madness, but sadly, the focus on growth (more clinics, more volume) without profit is how 99% of the profession is operating, and it is why there are so many tired business owners who are working until all hours of the morning with less and less to show for it.

It is important to remember that there is a big difference between growing, and growing profitably. Just ask General Motors, they were so busy getting big that they forgot to remember the purpose of a business is to actually be profitable.

THE "BOOM AND BUST" PHENOMENON

How else would you know that your clinic is absent of a predictable system for generating qualified leads? Well, you wouldn't be experiencing what I term the "boom and bust" situation of running a business.

Here's how this works: you get a sudden influx of new patients (all within a week or so), and that naturally keeps you too busy to do anything but treat them. It is great at the time, but what often happens after an influx of new patients is a "baron spell" with no names on the schedule, because you were too busy treating them to do any marketing (which keeps your schedule full).

There's no consideration of what that schedule is going to look like after the current batch of patients (who all arrived at once) have all finished their plan of care. The usual scenario is that right after they all get discharged from care, you look at next week's schedule, you realize it looks bare, and by the time you have done something about it, you notice that there has been three bad weeks with hardly any paying patients on your schedule. If that baron spell happens five or six times a year then you've lost a third of your earning potential. Sound familiar?

It used to happen to me all the time and it was costing me greatly.

If your goal is to grow a predictably profitable clinic, it pays to be aware of this "boom and bust" scenario in your schedule. If you are not careful you can spend your whole career with your numbers going up and down like a yoyo!

It is the period of time when you are in "bust" that will break you more than the "boom" periods will make you. This is why you need an automated marketing system: while you are busy treating patients you are constantly, and simultaneously, bringing in new leads and inquiries. The perfect situation is one where while you are working with one patient, another potential patient is filling out a form on your website, or is calling your clinic to inquire.

Instead of "boom and bust", we want to replace that with what I call the "constant, rhythmical acquisition of new patients", and this is the outcome you have to be aiming for if you want to grow profitably, year on year.

If the only time you are ever doing any marketing is when your schedule is empty, you will always have a limit as to the amount of growth you can see or profit you can make. What is more, to grow quickly you need leverage. Leverage is about getting more from doing less. For example, you're getting a steady supply of new inquiries whilst you are running your business, treating patients, or even while you are having dinner with the kids or are in bed sleeping at night.

Only by having a real marketing system will you ever get to this point in your business. I want you to **thrive** in business - not just **survive.**

MARKETING MISTAKE NUMBER #6: CHASING REFERRALS FROM DOCTORS

I've saved the best for last. So, why is marketing to the doctors a mistake? It's because statistically, mathematically, the odds of you being successful are stacked so far against you that it is almost impossible for you to have any chance of success.

Let me explain it with the help of a research study I came across a few years ago. Two very well respected guys in our field, namely "JM Fritz" and "JD Childs" wrote a study called "Primary Care Referral of Patients With Low Back Pain To Physical Therapy: Impact On Future Health Care Utilization And Costs" (*there's a link to the actual study in your resources PDF which you can get at www.paulgough.com/resources). The summary of what they found is basically this: despite the research showing that the cost of care and the speed at which the patients got better when patients are given a referral for physical therapy by a doctor, only 7% are actually given that referral.

Yes, just 7% of people of who are visiting their doctor with low-back pain are ever being given a referral for physical therapy. That outcome is despite clear evidence showing that it is the best path for them to take.

Let's take a look at what that means and how it applies to what I told you earlier in the chapter about the importance of focusing on the right target market. The whitepaper says that just 7% of people with low-back pain are being given a referral for physical therapy.

Now, first of all, the research tells you that physical therapy, and the benefits of what we do, is not all that understood by medical doctors or physicians (I think we all know this, but this is worse than I had thought…) Secondly, if doctors are not that confident about referring their patients to us, how can we possibly expect the patient to self-refer simply by seeing an ad that says "I'm an experienced and friendly physical therapist, call me today"?

It is madness to think they'll do it when so much confusion exists about what we do. Look at the situation more closely - on one hand, we have doctors who don't know what we do, and on the other, we have patients who visit us not knowing what we do.

At my clinic I can pretty much sum up how the conversation with the medical doctor will go (for these overlooked 93%), "it's your age", "rest it", "accept it" – or worse still, "here are some pills, come back in 6 weeks if it is no better".

Can you see the problem and where the chokepoint is in this profession? If patients don't know what we do, the only option is to educate them. How you do that is contained in this book.

YOUR BIG OPPORTUNITY

You might not be in the USA, and you might not specialize in low back pain (and so on and so on), but unless doctors have somehow, miraculously undergone specialized training on understanding what we really do and how we can help people – which is very unlikely – the same, or at least very similar thing, is going on in your town despite where you live.

The identity crisis that the profession has (or "lack of identity") is real, and it is making it very difficult to grow a private practice if you rely on the old-fashioned marketing methods. If just 7% of people are being given a referral for back pain in the US, the exact same number is not going to be too different for people with knee pain, neck pain etc., wherever you are.

Here's what this study is really telling you - for every 100 people who visit their doctor, 93 of them are still walking around with a problem. Only there's an additional problem now - the confusion or worry caused by not getting the help the patients expect from their doctor.

This next bit is important to understand too - given that these 93 people have been to their doctor and she did not mention physical therapy as an option, what are the chances of them ever making an appointment on their own? I'd say almost zero. Moreover, what are your chances of success with running a marketing campaign that is all about physical therapy and how experienced, or qualified, you are? Again, it is very slim.

No matter how good you say you are, no matter how friendly or professional you say you are, or how many years of qualifications you have, even how affordable your services might be – they are not calling you because they do not think you are the option they need.

Read that one again… they don't think you are the option they need. So there's now a choice:

1) You can get angry and irate, and you can ask why is our profession being overlooked by medical doctors?

Or

2) You can figure out how to get access to the 93% being overlooked and start helping them.

WHY CHASE AFTER A SMALL PIECE OF THE PIE – LET'S GET FAT!

7% is a very small number on its own. But, it gets even worse when you consider that every physical therapy clinic in your town wants a bite of that cake.

If there are only seven referrals up for grabs (for every 100 with back pain) and in an average town there's at least 4-5 clinics within a 10-12 mile radius that means that there is one, maximum two, referrals for each clinic.

With numbers so low it isn't a wonder that so many clinics are getting less and less referrals from doctors. These clinics relying on referrals from doctors are quite literally "cat-fighting" with each other for the crumbs of the pie. Why would you do that?

You do not get the success, the fulfillment, and the wealth you want from your practice by living off crumbs. People who live off crumbs are skinny. The people who live off the 93% leftover pie, get fat.

I want you to get fat. Very fat.

THE MILLION-DOLLAR QUESTION

In your town right now there are thousands of people wandering around (perhaps walking right by your clinic) with problems you can help them with. Most clinics are overlooking them however, if you focus on them, and if you use your marketing to communicate with them in a way that no one else is doing, you are going to get more successful very quickly.

And so the million-dollar question is this - how do you get access to the 93% of people who are currently walking around your town with a problem that you can solve for them, but who just currently do not consider you an option?

Well, all will be revealed in the upcoming pages of this book. And now that you have an understanding of why most marketing has failed in the past, as well as the opportunities that exist for you when you become clear on your perfect patient, once you fix your message, we can start exploring how you go about doing this.

As we move into the next chapter I will tell you my full backstory as well as how I turned my story into my own marketing system. I will also tell you how you can copy this to attract a huge number of people, people the likes of whom my competition was overlooking and who came to my clinic happy to pay in cash.

2

IF THIS CAN WORK IN A SOCIALIST FREE HEALTHCARE SYSTEM, CAN IT WORK FOR YOU?

I was born and raised in Hartlepool, a small town in the North East of England. I am the father of two beautiful boys and am the eldest of three children. After graduating from Northumbria University (in Newcastle, UK), I started my career as a physical therapist in the professional soccer industry. I worked for two top-flight, full time professional soccer teams in the English soccer league (Darlington and Middlesbrough FC), and I assumed I would be doing that job for my entire career.

FIVE YEARS AS A PHYSICAL THERAPIST IN PROFESSIONAL SOCCER

As a kid, watching or playing soccer was all I ever did, so landing a role in professional soccer was a dream job for me.

I was working with multi-million dollar soccer players, some of whom were the players I grew up watching on TV. I was learning from world-class doctors and even got to sit-in on just about every operation from a hernia, to a complicated ACL reconstruction. It was fascinating - and I was learning more in a month than I could have hoped to learn in 10 years working for a "mill-like" hospital system, which was my only other option at the time.

Game days were my favorite! Running on the pitch in front of thousands of fans was a buzz, and my biggest highlight was running on the pitch in my home town. I had grown up watching so many great players running onto this pitch, and now it was me! Actually, I was working for, (and wearing of the colors of), Darlington FC – the closest, biggest, and most hated rivals of my hometown, Hartlepool. Think Yankees and Red Socks. Manchester Utd and Liverpool.

Separated by just 25 miles, the fans of Darlington and Hartlepool hate each other, and, both sets of fans knew where I was from. I was the lad from Hartlepool working for Darlington. It took a long time for the fans of Darlington to accept me and even longer for the fans of Hartlepool to ever forgive me! I spent five years working with Darlington, a time which included a spell working with Middlesbrough FC, a team that were in the English Premier League at the time.

And I loved every minute of it – **until I didn't...**

I WAS BEING HELD BACK!

In the last season of working for the soccer clubs I was beginning to feel as though the role was holding me back from fulfilling my true potential - **my entrepreneurial potential.** At the same time as working for the club I had started to see one or two private patients from a spare room in my home, (as well at the stadium after the players had gone) and they would pay me cash for my services. This was my first taste of being in business, and, after a few months of doing this, I was building up a small, but regular patient database, and I was starting to make some decent money on the side.

At the same time, I was growing increasingly tired of being told by the soccer club when, and even worse, how to do my job. Ultimately I also got fed up of spending a lot of time away from home.

Life is great in pro-sport – but you are always on the road! What's more, I realized that my salary and earning potential had hit a ceiling. There wasn't much more to be earned from working in professional soccer than what I was getting at the time. I knew that if I was going to make the income that my skills deserved, and give my family a chance at a better life, I was going to have to take a risk on going it alone and starting my own business full time.

THE RISK OF STARTING MY OWN BUSINESS

So after five full years in employment I quit my high profile job in pro-soccer. It was incredibly risky and frightening, especially since I had a nice salary coming in from my soccer job each month and everyone was reminding me of that fact. My mother asked me this question many times, "are you sure you know what you are doing?"… Of course I didn't - it just felt wrong to stay.

However, what I was worried about was the fact that physical therapy is available freely in the UK. I wasn't confident about people paying privately (cash) for something they could get for free.

You might have heard of my competition – it is called the NHS (the National Health Service). It is one of the most well-known brands, and one of the largest employers on the entire planet. There isn't a single person living in Britain who doesn't know it exists, not to mention that one of the things freely given by the NHS is physical therapy There's no copay, no deductibles, no excess fee to pay – **it is free.**

I TOOK THE RISK!

It was very frightening. At first I had to acknowledge that what I was going to compete with was "free", but moreover that I was asking people to pay for my services out of pocket. Because remember, every time I asked them to pay $175 equivalent, **they had a free option.**

But I risked it, and I started the company that is known as Paul Gough Physio Rooms in 2007. I had no money. I had no experience. I had no business skills. And I certainly didn't have relationships with doctors or third party referrals. I was petrified when I first started out as I had no idea how I was going to pay my mortgage or put food on the table.

STARTING FROM A SPARE ROOM IN MY HOME!

I remember it like it was yesterday. The summer of 2007 was when I started Paul Gough Physio Rooms. I started from a spare room in my home in Hartlepool, and I had soon set up a second place - a rented room in a fitness facility located in a town about 25 miles away from Hartlepool called Darlington.

Right out of the gate I was a multi-clinic owner! I was living the dream. And to get going I did what everybody in our profession does – I made use of my friends and family network. I got going with a nice steady patient base; the word of mouth referrals were coming in. And, after a few months, I was approached by third party referrers ("worker's comp" type companies) who would start to refer people to me with injuries from accidents at work, or car-crash victims who needed physical therapy.

A few years later I was doing okay. I was surviving. I was making a living, but nothing amazing had happened and my profits had flat-lined. I've since discovered that this thing that I call the "new patient flat line" is something that happens to almost every business owner after about two years in. I speak about this in-depth in Episode 2 of my "Physical Therapy Business School" podcast (available on iTunes, or to download, at www.paulgough.com/podcast-002). Essentially it describes how and why physical therapy businesses get "stuck"…

"THE NEW PATIENT FLAT-LINE"

Here's how it goes:

For the first couple of years you work hard, you "hustle", you tell everyone you know about your new start-up and you make use of your friends and your family network. You most likely visit every gym or relevant fitness facility or club in the area. You are building momentum, and for the first two years your numbers rise steadily. You go from 5 visits per week, to 10, to 20 – and then you "flat-line".

You hit 20 visits a week, and no matter what you do, you just cannot seem get past it. Some weeks it's 22 visits, some weeks it's 18, but no matter how hard you try to really scale, you hit this **invisible ceiling** that you can't break through no matter what you do. In the weeks where your numbers drop, you hustle some more; you knock on more doors, or you hand out some fancy new flyers hoping to get some more patients coming to your clinic. And you do, but only just enough to take you back to where you were the week before which is about 20 or so visits.

What happens next is that you are too busy treating the patients that your latest "hustling" brought in – so, you forget to make time to continue to market your services. Inevitably, a few weeks later the numbers dip again so you go out and repeat the process. And so the cycle goes on, and on, **and on.**

It might be different numbers than the ones in this example, but the premise is the same. Your numbers drop, you hustle hard, and the numbers come back up to the same level as before. You are too busy servicing those patients to market for new ones, and, when the current crop of patients discharge the numbers drop again. There's never any huge drop, but at the same time there's never any real growth. It happens to 99% of business owners and sadly so many get stuck in this vicious cycle for about 25 years. It is frustrating, and what is needed is not more "hustle" or hard work – it is a completely new strategy.

This strategy needs to be one that is automated, **doing the marketing for you** while you are busy with patients or running the business.

Essentially, what I have just described is the same thing that happened to me. Different numbers, but that frustrating feeling of being stuck is exactly the same! At that point in my life I wasn't broke, but I wasn't rich either. And because of the cutbacks in the National Healthcare System around this time (right after the 2008 recession) few jobs were available in the system which meant that more therapists were setting up their own practices.

And because of the recession, insurance companies were making big cuts to their re-imbursement fees making it harder for me to make a profit. I remember e-mails would come in to the office from insurance companies, or workers comp agencies, telling us that a 30%/ 40% reduction in our fees was imminent. So I was in a situation where I was working twice as hard (to make the same money) and now there were more clinics than ever setting up against me. I had to work harder than ever, and the take home pay at the end was getting less and less. The situation wasn't great and was about to get worse…

MY HEART SCARE – AT THE AGE OF JUST 31!

This lack of profit was the least of my worries. **My health started to suffer…**

At the beginning of 2012 I was working so hard - literally 12, 13, 14, 15-hour days, trying to keep up with seeing more patients just to make the same profit. I'm a very "hands on" manual therapist as I come from a soccer background where I'd always have my hands on players, so I massaged hamstrings, did DTF massages on sprained ankle ligaments, and mobilized many stiff spinal vertebrae.

Manual therapy was my unique value proposition. I'd massage all-day long, I'd be stretching, I'd be doing everything myself without an assistant. And, I don't use machines. So at the end of the day my fingers and hands would be hurting so badly that I couldn't even use them to send a text message. It got to the point that when people sent me a text message, I could only *call* them back because I physically couldn't press the button on the phone to type out the message. It was that bad – **but it got worse…**

In 2012, I ended up in the Dr. Phillips Hospital, in Orlando. I suffered a suspected heart attack at the age of 31 while on holiday in Disneyland.

I was rushed to hospital just two days into to my holiday while walking around with my family at Sea World. I had noticed a problem a few weeks before travelling, so I went to see my local doctor in England, he told me it would be ok – I was to go on holiday and get some rest. But I wasn't ok. And even though I was on vacation I felt constantly stressed, anxious, and tense. I got to Orlando on one of the hottest days of the year – the heat was unbearable and making me constantly dehydrated.

On day two of the trip I noticed sharp pains in my chest, pain running down my arm, shallow breathing, and it literally felt like my heart was stopping and missing beats. I couldn't be having a heart attack, I was only 31, but I quickly found myself in the emergency room with a suspected heart attack.

Ironically, this was my first experience with the US health-care system and how it worked… I am used to walking out of hospital without having to do anything except say thank you, but this time I came out of the hospital with a bill of about $10,000. I couldn't believe it. It was enough to tip my heart back over the edge on its own. Even more ironically, this was my first time understanding the real value of a "cash pay patient": because I was a tourist, and I was paying in cash at the time of service, they applied a $6000 discount to my bill!

How nice of Dr. Phillips.

I left the hospital in the US and, with the doctor's permission, I flew back to the UK a few days later. When I got back to England, after all the tests, the doctors told me that my business had caused serious heart stress and that I had to make some changes. I was diagnosed, and still living with, an "ectopic heart-beat".

My heart was never missing a beat – it was actually adding a beat! I was living off adrenaline, and because of that too many electrical impulses were being sent to my heart. The pulses were causing my heart to do more work than it should be doing.

The effect of my condition resulted in the same symptoms as that of a heart-attack. However, they were only made worse by me thinking that I was having a heart attack. So my "heart" wasn't the problem – it was the symptom of a problem. I realized that the biggest cause of my problem was the fact that I was not in control of my practice and my life. Other people were.

The effect of my lifestyle was the irregular heart-beat caused by being in a state of constant angst, stress, and worry over my business. I was literally burned out! I was running around, and I was working way too hard, and all that whilst having no real say in what was going on in my business. Insurance companies were slashing rates, more clinics were setting up in competition against me, and I had no idea how to get out of it. It was felt like I was trapped in a nightmare.

Worrying constantly didn't help bring in the patients, and I knew that I really didn't have a way of growing or scaling my practice: I lacked an understanding of the one thing every successful business needs. That is, **a solid marketing system** to bring in my own steady stream of patients, so that I could run my business on my terms.

I COULDN'T SEE A WAY OUT

I kept looking at the situation I was facing, and with a huge free healthcare system as my main rival, I just kept thinking that no one in my town is going to want to pay in cash for this type of service – definitely not to the point that I could scale a business that could confidently end the dreadful payment terms I had with insurance companies and workers comp.

I felt that there was no option. It felt like there was never going to be a way out. But with my heart scare something had to give. The doctors said I had been given a huge wakeup call, and ultimately I was given an early warning to do something about it, or I'd risk ending up like many business owners whose heart-trouble is irreversible, or worse, **fatal.**

I considered walking away from my business many times, but I was too in love with it to ever go through with that. The only solution was to find a way to take back control.

THE PROBLEM WAS THAT I HAD NO MARKETING SKILLS

So, after the heart-scare I did a lot of soul-searching. I knew I had to do something different. But, I had no marketing skills! I had relied on patients being sent to my practice by insurance companies, and I wasn't very good at converting people to a cash-based service, nor was I confident at asking them to pay out of pocket. In the beginning I had spent what little money I had on marketing that didn't work, and if I did get calls they were usually from the one-hit-wonder type of patients who want the cheapest possible service.

I'd hear the typical lines like "I want to come and see you, but I can't afford you". "I would come and see you if I only had the money", and, "I'll need to cancel all my sessions, I found a cheaper option". I'd hear all of those excuses over and over again.

For a while I thought it was the only way. I assumed that I would be hearing those excuses for the rest of my career. But, thankfully, something called **"educational based marketing"** came into my life at the right time. This was a new way to market your practice and acquire new patients by adding value up-front so that they see the value in advance. It changed everything for me.

I was introduced to it at a seminar in London on a Monday, and being so impressed with what I was learning, I was on a flight to Chicago on the Wednesday. I got on that flight solely to attend another seminar just to learn more about educational based marketing.

At that time, my first son Harry, was just 4 weeks old. It was a pretty bold decision to fly out of London on a whim to attend a marketing conference in Chicago, but I've always believed that if you wait for all of your ducks to line up, or for the stars to align, you will be waiting for a long time. I've learned that the "the ducks never line up", and if something is important enough, it is worth doing today.

I knew that the marketing conference in Chicago was likely to teach me something I needed to know, and was possibly my only chance of walking away from the hassles and headaches I was getting from my business. So, I booked my tickets. I booked my flight and hotel, and I was off to a Super Marketing Conference for four days in Chicago to learn more about **education based marketing.**

What followed that seminar was a love affair with marketing – and Trans-Atlantic flying! I went to the conference and completely fell in love with learning about marketing. It was the answer to all my business problems. I could not get the information in my hands fast enough, and at one point I would travel to and fro between London and America at least once a month to attend as many seminars as I could! I knew I had found the keys to the vault and I couldn't get enough teaching to curb my appetite for it. I was spending half of my time in my office and the other half on a plane to a conference (or jet lagged). I was travelling to places like Dallas, Orlando, New Orleans, St. Louis, LA, Cleveland – anywhere that had an event that would teach me more about education based marketing and the systems I needed.

At times I was leaving the UK on a Thursday for a 2-day conference in somewhere like Texas, and I'd be back in the UK by Sunday afternoon with the information that I needed ready to implement it all on the Monday morning. It was a crazy couple of years in between flying, (and then implementing what I was learning), trying to treat patients, run my business, and, of course, spend quality time with my son.

I look back now and can confidently tell you that the lead generation education based marketing strategy is the one single strategy I've used to grow my physical therapy business. It made me go from a clinic that had me stuck, almost burnt out and losing money, to one a million-dollar plus equivalent practice that lets me travel the world with my family for weeks on end. And it happened in less than 13 months. It was a fast turnaround for me.

Every year since discovering this method the business has made me a healthy six-figure profit (without me working in it). I now have 18 staff running the business for me. And as I build my other two businesses, I simultaneously speak all over the world on the same topic as I am writing about today.

I also found time to write my first book, The Healthy Habit (www.thehealthyhabitbook.com also available on Amazon), and best of all, I've got a self-serving practice with 80% of its patients coming to us and paying in cash without any input from doctors. These patients are happy to pay significantly higher fees, too – meaning, we can operate a lean business, and make more money, despite seeing fewer patients. We also have significantly fewer expenses than most.

What do I mean by "self-serving"? It means we are in control. I decide how many patients come into my practice every single week by using the marketing systems I've got. If I want more patients, I spend more on marketing to put more patients into the system. If I don't, I stop. I can tell you precisely how many patients I will have every single week based on these marketing systems. It's that powerful.

I can see our schedule chock-full weeks in advance, and because we have people in the pipelines for making inquiries (from Group 2) we never have to worry about a "barren spell" or what to do if the numbers drop. If we see a dip, we go straight to the pipeline and look to convert more of them faster.

We are 100% in control of everything that is happening. We still get about 20% referrals coming from workers' comp or insurance – but, I call that the "gravy on top." If we get it, we get it. It's great. We don't particularly need it, but if we get it, as long as they are good payers – and they pay on time – then we will accept the referrals. But, we are not relying on them anymore and that is the difference that has made the change.

RECOGNIZED, TRUSTED AUTHORITY FIGURE IN MY TOWN!

The impact that this marketing strategy has had upon my life has reached well beyond just a better, more financially solid business. Not long after I started this type of marketing, I was approached by two local newspapers who asked me to be a weekly health expert in their publication.

Education based marketing is all about giving value and providing people with helpful information about how to make good decisions about their health. And so, when I was writing the ads to promote my clinic, the editors of the local newspapers liked what they saw. The style of the ads (which I'll teach you in chapter 8, "The Attraction System"), caught the attention of the editors, and two of them approached me and asked me to write weekly newspaper columns on the topic of health.

Ever since then I've written weekly newspaper columns in two of the big newspapers in my area (*I have provided an example of these newspaper columns in your resource pack that accompanies this book – get them at www.paulgough.com/resource). This provided, and still provides, free awareness of my clinic, and it also gave me the added bonus of positioning myself as the trusted authority – almost celebrity – healthcare expert in the North East. Imagine how easy it is to attract patients and raise your rates when you have this going on.

That awareness did this for me, and it can do the same for you.

MORE TIME TO TRAVEL THE WORLD WITH MY BOYS!

The justification for everything that I've done – all of the travel, the jet lag, and the money invested to get this marketing system working in my clinic – is that I now get to travel the world with my boys. My son Harry had been to Australia twice by the time he was 2, and as well as that, my boys have been to places like Disneyland, Washington D.C, New York City, LA, San Diego, Philadelphia, Denver, San Francisco, Miami, Dubai, and all across Europe too.

As a result of these systems by the time Harry was 4 he had been to 13 different states in the U.S. My youngest son, Tobias, is on this journey with me now too. Within two days of him being born we were at the passport office in the UK (we had to) and he was booked on a flight to California just 11 days later.

In the calendar year before writing this book, I spent a total of 22 weeks out of the UK, away from my practice, while it continued to run without me.

I am now free to pursue other business opportunities – Paul Gough Media LLC is a company that I set up in the US to continue providing marketing and business support to clinic owners all over the world. I get invited to attend and to speak at conferences around the globe – and of course, I found time in my day to write this book for you! (*Many of my keynotes appear on my "Physical Therapy Business School Podcast" that is available on iTunes and Android).

I've since been able to invest heavily in real estate and I was even able to buy two of the premises that my clinics operate from. I am now my own landlord, and as well as increasing my income, I am building lasting wealth for my family. Having an automated marketing system has made all of this possible for my family and I, and I am delighted to be able to share that system with you as we work through this book together.

Your goal might not be to spend 20 weeks of the year away with your kids - but whatever your goal is, I know that following the system outlined in this book is going to help you achieve it.

Anyhow, now that I have told you my story and how I came to find the solution to my business (and health) problems, let's get started on the system that will show you how to maximize the return on investment (ROI) of your time and money…

3

HOW TO 10X YOUR PROFIT USING MARKETING

Quick question: do you want "more new patients"? Or do you want "more new patients that are happy to pay higher prices, who respect what you say and do for them, and are willing and able to pay upfront?"… Which would mean that you can make more profit, get paid faster, and go home earlier each day? If your choice is the latter, then you will love this chapter of the book.

You see, marketing (Paul Style!) is not just about getting more new patients. What I have learned, and what I will teach you in this book, is that business success, wealth, lifestyle, or prosperity – whatever it is you are looking for – is not found in simply getting a higher volume of patients. That is great for the ego, but not always great for your bank balance or your stress levels.

Marketing "Paul Style" is 100% about getting more calls from the right patients who are a pleasure to work with, are happy to pay your much deserved higher fees, and who preferably pay with crisp, fresh dollar bills from the ATM machine.

I can show you lots of clinics, with lots of patients coming through the doors, but those same clinic owners are often devoid of any cash, burned out, stressed out, and always missing out on their kids. I am going to assume that this is not what you want. The most important "P" in your business is PROFIT, and with that said, here are seven of the best ways to use your marketing to ensure that you get a lot more money.

And what you will soon see is that when you use your marketing (Paul Style!) for any, or all of these reasons below, it is so much easier to be successful with it. You'll be growing your clinic on your terms, outside of the insurance system, and without needing referrals from doctors. These are important distinctions that many business owners never even consider, and marketing can significantly stack the odds of success in your favor. For example…

1. SEPARATE YOURSELF FROM "MILL LIKE" PHYSICAL THERAPY CLINICS

If you are a new clinic trying to get profitable quickly, or an established clinic with a small marketing budget trying to fight against the big corporate "Mill PT Clinics", it can seem an almost impossible task when you look towards the future. But remember, David did beat Goliath. And you can beat the bigger clinics and hospital systems, too. But not if you try to play them at their own marketing game, one which usually involves spending a lot of money on "image ads" that promote logos, or show pictures of two smiley, happy people looking back at each other. All these adverts do is try to insinuate that the health and happiness being portrayed in the image is thanks to the clinic doing the advertising.

This is not great advertising. It is a sloth-like use of corporate money, and I assure you if the people who were running the ads had to put up their own money (like you and I do), they would not be doing it.

The good news is that their poor marketing strategy is your biggest advantage. It gives you an easy path to positioning yourself as genuinely different in the community you serve, and it also gives you an easy path to connecting with more of the ideal types of patients you want to serve.

Now, before I go any further, if you are not familiar with the term 'Mill PT Clinic", it is typically used to describe the types of corporate clinics that care more about volume than quality of care. They see their patients as "bill-able units", and their staff as "units of production". A typical day for a physical therapist working at a "Mill PT Clinic" could involve seeing up to as many as 50 patients per day. No exaggeration. They are big and ugly, and the care is dreadful. It is not the fault of the therapist, rather it is 100% the fault of the corporate directors and bean counters who care more about profits than their patients getting the time and attention that they really want and deserve. These clinics have huge ad budgets, and their marketing departments love to waste money by blanketing the newspapers, motorway billboards, or radio and TV stations in your town (as well as buy out local doctor offices), and it is easy to feel as though their presence is drowning you out.

But here's where this gets fun - the marketing that these types of companies do is almost as bad as the care they provide – it is awful (and that is me being respectful). They rely heavily upon mass advertising, and focus more on being seen than creating a deep and lasting impact with the people who see their message. They don't care who sees it so long as they are seen. It is 'hit and run' style advertising, and it only works for the big, stuffy, corporate clinics because they have so much money to waste. <u>There's no thought going into who the patient is or the problems they are living with</u>. It is very "intrinsic", all about the clinic and not about the patient.

You can instantly spot their ads - they will say something like "your health, our hands", or "a healthier you", or even something terrible like "the outcome you want, the care you deserve". The only thing they care about is how nice the ad looks. It is mass appeal marketing at its worst, and their goal is to get in front of the "ready to buy now" type of patient (Group 1, explained in chapter 1). That is, the small 3% of people in any town who are actively considering buying physical therapy.

And that is why I can confidently tell you that these big clinics are not something to be worrying over. You might think that you are in competition with these clinics, but you are not. Sure, you provide a service under the same name, but if you market in the way that I am teaching you, you will be marketing to a completely different pocket of people – the people in Group 2; the ones who need what you provide and who just need to see a little more from you so that they can hire you.

The people in Group 2 (the likes of Mary and Christine from chapter 1) are never going to go and see the big mill-like clinics – they don't know enough to confidently do it. And you and I know full well that the mill clinics are not going to take the time to help them make the right decision about their health.

2. GET MORE COMMITTED PATIENTS

Everyone is on a journey. Your journey building your business may just be starting. You may have been in business for 20 years already and are looking to go in a completely new direction. If you're just setting up, you are likely to be reading this book full of optimism and hope, motivated by the anticipation of good things that are to come for you. You are moving towards pleasure. Alternatively, if you've been in business for 20 years, chances are you feel stuck and are frustrated in your current predicament, and your motivation is to move away from the pain. Either way, you're on a journey, and you will make decisions at different speeds and for different reasons.

Your patients are doing that too. That journey for them most likely started weeks, months, years, perhaps even decades before they ever saw your ad, your clinic, or ever contemplated getting some help from you. This understanding of the "journey" is not something we are taught in school and most of us have been led to believe that people are literally just waking up one morning and calling their doctor the moment they are in any discomfort. They are not.

Think about all of the subjective assessments that you've ever done and you've asked the question, "how long has it been going on?" When was the last time they told you, "oh, it started just yesterday". For most of them the story started a long time ago. In between the start of the problem and the patient's decision to do something was the agony of deciding what to do about it.

"I WISH I'D CALLED YOU 12 MONTHS AGO – WHEN I FIRST SAW YOUR WEBSITE"

Now, all of this started to make sense to me after a conversation I had with a patient who came to see me – he had a long-standing neck problem. After the very first session he told me something that has stuck with me forever, and perhaps even changed my understanding of what I needed to do with my marketing. He had been suffering with neck pain and stiffness for about 3 years and he told me straight after that first session was over, "I wish I had come and seen you 12 months ago when I first looked at your website".

I couldn't believe what I was hearing. I replied, "you mean it took you an entire year to come and see me after you first found out about me?" He was a little sheepish and said that he knew he needed to do something, it was just that "some days it was worse than others", and on the better days he would convince himself that it was "going to be ok, so there was no point in calling", just incase he was wasting his time and money.

This indecision went on for 12 months until he finally realized that it wasn't going to go away on its own and he had to do something about it, i.e. come and see me. You might think "great, he came back to see you", but the reality is I was very lucky that he remembered who I was, as he saw my website a whole 12 months before the visit. Most people cannot remember what they had for breakfast this morning, never mind what website they were on 12 months ago!

This type of thing is, and will be happening to you right now, and when it comes to making the decision it is quite literally pot luck as to which physical therapy clinic will get the patient's call. That might be how some businesses want to live, but being at the mercy of a Google Free Business listing search it is not my idea of how you grow a sustainably profitable business. It is how you have a lot of sleepless nights, how you end up a commodity, and why you would struggle to ever charge enough to make going into business actually worthwhile.

The big lesson I learned from that conversation was the realization that everyone I was speaking to had some form of "I knew I needed to do something about this earlier – I just didn't know what". It became obvious that this was the rule and not the exception, so I decided to build my marketing system to factor this indecision in. The majority of people out there who have problems we can solve have some bad days followed by some good days, and every night they go to bed they secretly believe that tomorrow will be the day they wake up cured. When they don't wake up with the pain miraculously gone, they hope it will be by tomorrow - and so on, and so on, and so on.

3. CREATE "LIFERS" (HIGH VALUE, REPEAT PATIENTS)

When you stop and think about it, the real reason that many people are living with chronic pain today is simply because they did not know how to make a good decision when they needed to. They may have chosen to ignore the, pain, mask it with pills, not follow through on the medical person's advice given at the time, accept it, pass it off as an "age thing", or they may just think it is a genetic issue that they have to live with because everyone else in their family does.

Either way, the person now living with a 10-year history of back pain did not make a good decision. When you look at it from that angle, is there anything more important in a health-care clinic than getting your marketing system right? And wouldn't you if you can be the person who helps someone reverse a bad decision (to do nothing or keep taking pills), and it is going to be very impactful for your clinic profits? They are going to love you forever (repeat, lifelong business) if you can take them from thinking that "nothing can be done" to being active and mobile again, or even living free from painkillers.

When you use your marketing to attract and then help these people who had quite literally "given up hope", there is no way that they are going to see another physical therapist other than you ever again. This is one of the reasons we get so many repeat patients – "lifers" – who just come back and see us time and time again. Not only that, they bring their friends and families too because they credit us with helping them achieve something that everyone else told them couldn't be achieved.

In reality, all we did was use our marketing to show them that it was possible, and with that they gave us the opportunity to do what we do best. There's no shortage of people with money out there, and they have problems that you can solve. But, there is a shortage of people out there who seem to want to hand it over in exchange for a solution from a physical therapist. Why is that I wonder? Could it be that we just do not do a good enough job of communicating what we can actually do for people and how we can help them? I think so.

CLEARING UP THE "BS" ABOUT WHY IT'S "WRONG" TO MARKET IN HEALTHCARE

And that's why it makes me laugh when I hear some people in our profession say that healthcare professionals "should not be marketing", or that "it is wrong to market to patients in pain". Anyone suggesting this is being ignorant and arrogant as to how marketing actually works.

They live closed off from ever discovering how valuable proper marketing can be in enhancing the relationship you have with your patients. What's more, these people have completely misunderstood how people really need to be helped (at the point of decision), neither do they understand what marketing actually is.

Clinicians often see marketing as "bad" simply because they think it detracts from the superior skill set (that they think they have); they've been brain-washed into thinking that skill set is all that's required. Their self-worth is often tied to their own perceived level of skill and heaven forbid anyone comes along and is more successful simply by having a better website or marketing message.

The person who thinks that "marketing is wrong" is usually the one who is more concerned about credentials and qualifications (ego!). His head is stuck too far up his own "ass" to ever get it out and see that marketing's only job is to ensure that those skills, and those credentials, are actually utilized. In that respect, and if you are clinically skilled, marketing is your best friend. And you should be embracing it as the vehicle that is going to put you in front of more people who you can help.

I don't know about you, but I am in business to help people, and over the years I've realized that the only way that I can help people is if they actually know I exist. I know a lot of clinicians with a lot of skills who will not market themselves and as a result, have empty schedules and equally empty bank balances. Do not copy their ignorant ways of thinking about marketing. The fact remains that the company with the best marketing always wins. Besides, all those companies that you consider to be great – how did you hear about them in the first place?...

4. SELL ONLY WHAT THEY WANT TO BUY

Finding out early what your prospective patients want to pay for is pretty important. It allows you to sell them what they want, instead of what you think they need. No one likes to be sold to – but, they love to buy. So how about you use your marketing to find out exactly what they want?

The biggest roadblock that many physical therapists in business hit is in selling something that the patient does not want to buy, i.e. "pain relief". Just because they are in pain does not mean that they want to pay to have it eased – despite what we might think. The easiest way to create a business where more people want to buy more from you is to simply ask them what it is they want. As in, use your marketing to find out for certain and have them prove it to you with their actions.

After years of marketing my clinic directly to the public (and spending $100,000's to learn this lesson) I can confidently tell you what my patients do not want is physical therapy. How do I know that people do not want to pay for physical therapy? I asked them in many newspapers, on Facebook, and in postcard and leaflet campaigns. I ran these campaigns to advertise the fact that I am a "Friendly and Experienced Physical Therapy Clinic", and in them I asked the patients to "call and book an appointment at my practice". Here's the painful lesson I learned: no matter how much I spent, or how big and fancy the ad or promotion was, I hardly ever got any response from a typical ad that said "I'm a Physical Therapist, call today".

However, when I used my marketing to ask the same people (reading the same newspaper or seeing me on Facebook) if they wanted help with things like "maintaining independence", "keeping active and mobile", or, "living a life without pills", (which meant they could also stay out of the doctor's office), **they called in droves.**

What the people in my community were telling me was that they **wanted the outcome,** not my service or skills needed to get it. It will be the same in your community too no matter where you live. In the early stages, it is smart to use your marketing to test different messages and to promise different outcomes, so you can clearly see which one resonates the most. I notice the difference even when I switch between my marketing message being about "getting off pills" or "avoiding surgery". Understanding this also helps you at the point of conversion and ensures compliance. For example if I run an ad that says, "I'll help you get off pills", then I know that my entire communication and plan of care has to be matched up against achieving **that** outcome. After all, that is why they called in the first place.

The minute I start talking about "giving them great service", I dilute the meaning of what I will be doing for them and ultimately what they are paying for. That is when they drop off the schedule. Sell them what they want to buy and they'll spend more money with you. Marketing is pivotal to figuring this all out, and ultimately, it is the key to higher profits.

5. MORE TRUST = MORE HAPPY PATIENTS (SPENDING MORE $$$ WITH YOU)

Something that is an absolute pre-requisite for your success in business is 'trust'. Said differently, the no.1 reason that people do not buy from you is because there is a **lack** of trust. If you do not build it, patients will definitely not come. However, the good news is that there is a way to build more trust using your marketing. This for me is one of the biggest advantages in marketing, and it is definitely the most overlooked - it points directly to why you must have a marketing system in place at your clinic.

Trust is so important in your business, because people fear and hate the prospect of making the wrong decision. Because of this, they become more focused on avoiding a bad decision than actually working out how to make a good decision. They become risk averse. By the time people hit 40 they have made so many bad decisions they will do anything to avoid the consequence of getting another one wrong. "Buyers' regret" is real – it's a chemical called "cortisol" that flows through your body when you do something that you later regret, or doesn't give you the outcome that you wanted. It is not pleasant, and unbeknownst to them, most people are spending their lives in a perpetual state of procrastination simply by trying to avoid more of this chemical.

The solution is to build "trust" in the patient's relationship with you, and however long that takes to achieve make sure it is done so well, so thoroughly, that he feels it is almost impossible to see hiring you as a bad decision. My goal is to have my prospects arrive in a "trust matured" state, whereby at the time they arrive at my clinic, committed and already bought in to what we can do for them, there is no question about whether or not we are the right provider.

It is essential that you have enough of these "trust matured" patients wanting to hire you, otherwise you will always be dealing with people who are not wanting to pay your fees, always resisting the prescription of care, and always telling you that they will need to speak to their insurance first.

The trust building process is not just about fostering trust in you or physical therapy, it's not even about the outcome, it is largely about the patient building trust in themselves and in their own ability to make a good decision. The only solution to this issue is to provide information so that they can feel confident in the decision to hire you as ultimately, information acts as the gateway to better decisions.

If you stop and think about it, most of the bad decisions that you made happened because you probably didn't do your homework. You didn't request information on the subject beforehand, and instead, you made an emotional decision to act simply because it felt right. So, the antidote to the patient feeling like they could come out the other side having made a wrong decision is to bridge the gap with information. In chapter 6, I will show you precisely how to create the information needed to build that trust.

6. MORE VISITS (AT HIGHER PRICES)

It is hard to grow a profitable business if you are forever attracting "ones-ey, twos-ey" type of patients. What does that mean? It means that the hardest part of growing a business is getting the customer in the first place, and if they are only having one or two sessions with you it is impossible to make a profit. The revenue from one or two sessions barely covers the cost of getting them in the door.

"We fix your pain", or "we get you out of pain fast", are great slogans, but they will not attract the types of patients that will want to pay the type money, and make the type of commitment you will need in order to grow your business. First of all most people are not in that much pain, and even if they are, they've probably called someone by now. Even if you get them, they'll be gone after two or three sessions when the pain is gone. But what about the muscle weakness, balance problems, and other joints and muscles that have been affected? All those need some attention (and you need to be paid to do it) but if you only promise to solve their pain then that is all they will want to pay for, not the other issues that need addressing.

However, if you use your marketing to show how you can solve problems that are much more deep-rooted than just "pain", then you will bring patients to your clinic who value what you do enough to want to pay for it. These problems could be for example, an inability to walk with a husband along the beach and enjoy the great feeling that exercise brings, or even the ability to look after the grandkids during the day, able to pick them up with ease. And that is the "nirvana" that we have to be shooting for - attracting patients who value you enough to want to pay for it. It is your marketing message that makes this happen, and it can ultimately affect your profitability.

LESS HASSLE AND MORE PROFIT

My clinic now sees fewer new patients than it did 5 years ago – but, we make more profit. This is no coincidence that it coincided with a switch in our marketing from "book now if you are in pain", to, "if you are frustrated with having to rely upon pills, call me". What I do these days is essentially **solve the issue that the first problem creates.**

Here are a couple of other examples of what I mean by that, as well as how you might adopt it:

- Is a person who has recently had a stroke looking for a new physical therapist, or are they worrying over whether they will ever be able to be independent again? Are they desperately wanting an additional 10% or 20% improvement in the quality of their life? The latter two questions are key – and that is what should be communicated in your marketing message

- If you are talking to parents of children with disabilities, do you think they want another physical therapist? Or, do they want to be 100% certain that they are giving their child the best possible opportunity to access the best care that medicine can currently provide? The major problem that the disability CREATES is a parent worried over whether she is doing her best for the child.

- It is the same with back pain; is the patient more concerned about chronic low back pain, or worried about the consequence of a lifetime depending on pills?

In all of these cases, it is "the problem that the problem creates" that is the real suffering.

It is mostly to do with the patient being worried, frustrated, skeptical, frightened, or even unsure about the future. These are very painful states to be in, and if you can change your marketing to show that you can solve these problems, you're going to be a lot more successful than just telling people how many qualifications you have or that you can fix low back pain.

7. SHOWING VALUE UPFRONT (ALLOWS YOU TO RAISE YOUR RATES FREQUENTLY)

"Showing value up front" is my favorite use of marketing, and if you use marketing for this, it will really separate you from all of your competition – and it will let you raise your rates. The buzz words in our profession right now are "show them the value" – meaning, if you want to be more successful in private practice then you have to show people proof of the quality you will bring to their lives (in exchange for the time and money they will have to give up). When is the best time to show them proof of value? It is in advance of them having to actually pay you any money.

Think about it, for most business owners the proof of value only begins when the credit card or insurance number is handed over and the clinical skills come out. Value is a concept that is open to many different definitions and interpretations, yet it is affected only by the perception of the BENEFITS that the patient thinks he is going to receive (as discussed in further detail in chapter 4). These benefits are all influenced by your marketing, and therefore showing more of those benefits starts with understanding what the person you are trying to help actually values.

What they value most is the **end outcome.** In my clinic's case, that outcome could be more independence, a more active lifestyle, a life free from pills, or a life suited to playing with their grandkids for longer. When you truly understand what the outcome is your perfect patients are looking for, you can start to communicate this in your external marketing. You want to instantly show the value of what you can do for them before they even arrive at your clinic.

How do you know if you are showing value in your marketing? It's easy – you will be able to raise your prices whenever you feel like it. I'm serious too. I've had many of my Accelerator Program students raise their rates as much as three times in one calendar year, as a result of showing value upfront with their marketing. And I'm not just talking about a measly $5 rise on the first of January like every other broke business owner does. I'm talking $50, $75, even $100 raises with little (if any) pushback. One Accelerator Method student that springs to mind is Carrie Jose (of CJ Physical Therapy and Wellness, Portsmouth, NH) – she seems to raise her rates every time we speak! Before Accelerator, she was stuck charging just $150 per visit, thinking that no-one would ever pay anything more than that in "little-old Portsmouth." How wrong she was - at the time of writing this book Carrie is charging $295 per visit. Way to give yourself a pay rise!

A lack of proof of value up front is the primary reason that so many physical therapists struggle to raise prices. And that's a shame, because the fastest way to boost profits is to increase the prices.

At my clinic, as soon as we get busier than we can handle, my go-to strategy is not to employ a new therapist to cope with the demand, but to raise the rates to fend off demand! Employing staff comes with headaches and hassles – raising rates is fun and profitable. I like raising rates. The increase is all mine and I get to spend the difference on my kids and doing nice things with my family.

Now that you see this is about a lot more than just "more new patients", let's look at why your marketing system is the secret to attracting all of the high value, cash-paying patients.

4

HOW TO ATTRACT PATIENTS HAPPY TO PAY CASH

Every single one of us is in business to make a profit, right? Otherwise what's the point? Sure, you want to help people and serve them well, but you could have worked for someone else all your career if that is all you wanted to do.

Profit is very important. But I think there's a tendency for physical therapy business owners to think that, "if I just get more patients", everything will be ok. It's as if volume will solve every problem they've got. That isn't always the case. Ultimately, the purpose of a business is to turn your assets (of which your marketing system is one) into **revenue,** turn your revenue into **profit,** and your profit into **cash** (so that you can cover the running costs that the business incurs and can have the take home a salary you deserve).

If you do not focus on profit and having cash in the bank, you'll struggle and will eventually go out of business. It's that simple.

Attracting more cash pay patients solves both of those problems in one go. More profit – and, more cash in the bank. It's why I am such a big advocate of you getting a load more cash patients through your doors. With insurance reimbursements dropping year on year, what other option is there?

I think the phrase "skate to where the puck is going – not where it has been" sums up the situation perfectly. And if you are not chasing the puck in the direction of a significant amount of cash pay, then you are likely to find yourself with a business that might be growing but is getting less profitable as repayments drop. Owning a business like that is going to make you very tired, stressed, and always feeling like you have to work harder just to make the same money. Can you relate?

As we move through this chapter together I am going to share with you the exact strategy I used; the one that allowed me to be able to move away from relying mostly upon insurance based patients – being trapped inside of the system – to a now mostly cash pay clinic that is more profitable and **sees less** patients. I will be sharing with you precisely how I was able to market my practice to make it more attractive to higher value, cash-pay patients, and I'll let you in on the no.1 secret to cash pay marketing success that I am glad I discovered so early on.

THE MOST PROFITABLE MOVE I MADE IN BUSINESS

Switching my clinic's marketing to focus on cash pay patients was liberating for me – to exit the insurance system was easily the smartest and most profitable decision I ever made. I would recommend it to anyone. However, if you are mostly an insurance-based clinic as you read this, I am NOT suggesting that you immediately end all of the contracts you have with insurance companies. That would be reckless. However, what I am suggesting is that you give at least some thought to the impact that it would have on your business profits if you dropped 20% of the worst payers and replaced $85 reimbursements, (that take weeks to arrive in your bank) with $250 "fee for service" cash pay patients instead who either pay upfront or as they go.

I've got Accelerator Method students all over the USA who have done exactly that. Let me introduce you to one of them, Kim Gladfelter of Physio-Fit in San Jose, Ca. Kim's average reimbursement from the insurance companies was something like $85, and her running costs were something like $82 per hour. It was almost impossible for Kim to sustain running a business on margins so thin. Twelve months after implementing the Accelerator system in her practice, she had dropped many of those crappy insurance companies and swapped $85 reimbursements with cash-pay rates closer to $200 per visit. Not only is Kim significantly more profitable, her practice is seeing fewer patients and she also has a much better cash flow. Win-win.

Now, here's a key point: it is important to have both profit and cash flow if you want to grow a sustainable business. I know a lot of insurance-based clinics who are "profitable" on paper, but never have any money. They are spending it on expenses faster than they are getting paid, living month to month hoping that the big check will arrive on time, sweating that all claims will get approved. All it takes is one screw up by the billing company you hired and you are in the hole, struggling to pay the wages at the end of the month. All of those problems disappear when you are getting paid at the time of service, or even better, when you're paid up front for a 10-session plan of care.

When it comes to building a physical therapy clinic, cash really is "king".

ULTIMATELY, WE ARE ALL IN THE CASH PAY BUSINESS THESE DAYS

Here's something else to consider; whether or not you want to drop some of those crappy insurance companies and bring in more cash pay patients with your direct marketing, what you must factor in is that as the cost of healthcare rises, technically you are already in the "cash pay" business.

Here's what I mean: anytime anyone is self-funding a significant chunk of their treatment with you, their expectations and demands have changed – and so must you.

Think about it, if you are asking patients to pay $50 copay twice per week for four weeks, it means they are paying you $400 in cash out of their own pocket. If your patients are having to pay hundreds of dollars in cash for your services to cover copay, or break into a $2000 deductible in January to start treatment with you, then you are **already** in need of having to know how to market, sell, and communicate in a different way just to service the patients you already have.

If you are in Canada and the patient's insurance limit is $500, and they need more sessions to get their outcome once that limit is hit, the total of another three sessions might be $250 or more. They have to pay you in cash out of their own pocket to do that. You too, are already in the cash pay business. You too, are in need of a completely new way to encourage people to **understand why they need to pay it.**

If you are in the UK and you are still working with insurance companies or medical agencies, but the patient has a £200 excess on their policy, you are asking them to pay in cash to start the treatment. Obviously they have an alternative to that payment with the free NHS physiotherapy dept., so if you do not market and speak to them from the get-go, and in a way that they can understand and in a way that will help them know why they should pay that £200 to you - then they simply won't.

You too, are already in the cash pay business.

The same is happening in Australia, New Zealand, and all over Europe. One way or another, every person reading this book is likely to be in the cash pay business either completely or partly. Either way, though, you are likely heading closer to the model of having more people pay in cash than not, so it pays to know how to do it right.

WHAT IS THE DIFFERENCE BETWEEN CASH PAY AND TRADITIONAL INSURANCE BASED CLINICS?

It is funny, because if you asked a cash pay clinic owner what they believe the difference is between them and an insurance based clinic, they'd likely tell you it is a "higher level of service", the fact that they provide "one-one-one care", or that their 'skills' are somehow better, and that is how they can justify the extra cost…

And yet, if you ask an insurance-based business owner that same question, he will also tell you that he provides great service with unrivalled care, that he has the best skills, and that group sessions are what patients want.

It should be understood that they are both offering essentially the same thing, despite each owner believing that his is a slightly better version. The problem is all of those things being mentioned are "features" of the service being offered (your level of service and skills). Features sound great, but if you want to get more cash patients into your clinic, the difference will not be in how great you explain the features. Why? Because the price point that you are asking people to pay, is sometimes as much as $100-$200 more. It is way too big of a leap for a 'slightly better' feature. The patient is not going to pay that much extra for a little bit more of essentially the same thing. The only thing that they will pay more for is the promise of a different outcome (the benefits your business offers as a result of treatment).

Most business owners are naïve to the fact that when it comes to solving their problems, which are associated with lower reimbursements and rising push back to patient contributions, **it is not a slightly better version of the same thing that patients want**, it is the promise of something different.

This is a point I rose recently when I was invited to speak at the American Physical Therapy Association's (Private Practice Section) Annual Conference in Chicago. This event was attended by 10,000 private practice owners, and I told all of them that their biggest problem was NOT lower repayments or patient compliance since costs have gone up, but that it is actually in the way that they see the problem...

See, the implications for how you must speak to and market to people who are making a bigger commitment with you, (by paying in cash and with larger sums), are huge. And yet, it never ceases to amaze me how most physical therapists are still talking to, marketing to, and selling to their patients in the exact same way that they did when the cost of health care was 10x less than it is today.

As I explained to the physical therapists in the room with me that day, our profession has taken the approach that all of the problems, which are associated with the rising cost of healthcare, can be solved by 'more research and better skills'.

Now of course, I understand why they would think like this. After all, there's the not-so-small matter of student loans that were borrowed in conjunction with the guarantee and promise of what better skills would do for us. But the problem is the patient doesn't care about slightly better skills. At the point of deciding to hire a physical therapist, all she cares about is getting the **outcome** which will justify the significantly higher cost.

Sure the skills help achieve the outcome, but I honestly don't believe that many physical therapists reading this book have a problem achieving the outcome. Do you?

The problem is getting in front of enough patients who will be happy to pay for allowing a physical therapist to achieve the outcome. **Big difference.**

So, what is needed to help private practices survive is not more research or more clinical skills for the sake it. No, instead it's a much better way of communicating with patients. We need to spell it out to them that we know how to help them achieve their desired outcome in a way that is better than any other option they have.

That, by the way, is the no.1 job of your marketing.

Could it be that the real reason many clinics are struggling right now is because they don't do any marketing… or they "half-ass" what they do? It is highly likely.

THE NO.1 SECRET TO CASH PAY MARKETING SUCCESS

Everything that I have just told you above is advice that I have heeded myself. It is not always pleasant, but I prescribe and swallow my own medicine.

My clinic is now mostly "cash pay". We switched our model from being 80% reliant upon medical agencies, lawyers, and other third party referrers, thus having about 20% cash pay (in 2011), to now being 80% cash pay and 20% third party referrals. We have tipped the business on its head, and the effect of it has been stunning.

Moving out of the system that had me trapped and struggling to make a profit (whilst relying on low-reimbursements), and into a model that has me in control of what we charge, as well as how many sessions we can see patients for, was easily the best and most profitable decision of my business career to date.

I've learned a lot of lessons about how to do it, and it all started by me asking a better question than just, "how do I get more cash patients?" Here's a much better question… one that when answered correctly will solve the profit problem that most physical therapists currently have:

> **"How do you get someone to pay cash (or out of pocket) for something that is <u>easily</u> and <u>freely</u> available to them for <u>cheaper</u> elsewhere?"**

If you re-read that sentence again, you'll see that the question really sums up the situation that you and I are facing.

Basically, we are asking people to pay more, perhaps even the full payment in cash. We're asking them to pay for something, that because of insurance or free national health care (and not forgetting other, more cheaper providers like massage therapists and personal trainers who are often promising the same outcome), can now be freely and easily found (because of Google and the Internet).

It is not the "million dollar question", no, this one is the **"multi-million dollar question"**… "How do you get more of your traditional insurance-type patients (or people in a country with free health care) to pay for your services with their own money?"

Want to know the answer? I'm about to reveal it to you…

HOW TO MAKE THEM HAPPY TO PAY IN CASH

The answer is to **focus on the difference they have to pay for the difference you can make.**

Now let me explain that in more detail - really, when all is said and done, all patients want to know is "what is the difference (i.e. $50 or $100) I have to pay, and how will you (the more expensive provider) make that difference worthwhile and justifiable?"

The answer is **not** to do what I've seen a lot of clinic owners do, which is perform a long winded mathematical equation in front of them. Don't painstakingly attempt to do that while they're with you, just because you will be able to "help them achieve their outcome in less sessions", than the seemingly cheaper insurance provider who will make them come for more sessions than you… Because the patient will ultimately end up paying less!

It is much simpler than that. Besides, that tactic is dreadful – it **attracts the wrong type of patient** as it always comes back to "cost". They are still going to be choosing you because you are cheaper, and **we do not want** someone to choose you just because you are cheaper.

That is not a good place to get compliance for a plan of care you are about to prescribe.

We want them to choose you because you offer more value. This is the only thing that they should be allowed to judge you on, because broadly speaking, what most people really want more than "cheap", is value. And if you do not provide clear evidence of value – then of course they will always go with the cheaper provider. And rightly so.

THE VALUE EQUATION: VALUE = BENEFITS / PRICE

So, let's talk about value. Looking specifically at how you can offer more of it to get more lucrative, cash paying patients for your clinic.

Value is what the patient wants, right? Value is what you bring to a patient's life as a result of what you do for her using your skills. Value is what she gets in exchange for her time and money. Ultimately, value is the difference that you will make to that person's life. It makes paying the price (in both time and money) worthwhile.

So then the next question to ask is this - "how does the patient get to decide what this thing called "value" actually is?"...

Well, it's as simple as this - **value is determined by the benefits you bring, divided by the price the patient has to pay** - in our case, the outcome you provide to the patient divided by the total cost of all the sessions needed to achieve it.

Now, because of the way the above value equation works, you can very easily add more value to a patient's life by simply lowering the price of your service. And sadly, this is what most cash pay clinics do - they are naïve as to how the value equation can be altered in a different way.

But I am going to assume that dropping your fees is not the way that you want to bring more value. Am I right? If so, lets both work through the value equation; I'll show you how you can alter the value the patient received by modifying the benefits, not just lowering the price…

Example 1: Let's say there's a typical cash pay clinic in your town. The marketing message is about "easing pain fast" with "great service" (standard stuff that most rookie marketers boast about). What you should know is that this marketing message – in this case, the "friendly service" and the promise of "easing pain fast" – is actually also the benefit that they are promising to anyone who hires them.

In this hypothetical example, there is a reasonable amount of benefits being promised, so let's apply a figure to it of 450 units of benefits that will be felt by the patient overall when hiring this clinic[1] (this figure will become relevant as you read on). And, let's say the clinic is charging is $150 per session to get those benefits. That means the value that this clinic is bringing has a numerical value of 3 (450/150).

So, if this cash pay clinic wanted to add more value they could drop the price to $100, and, for the same benefits ("friendly service and easing pain"), the patient is now getting a value score of 4.5 (450/100).

The patient is now getting more value, but the clinic owner is getting paid less. That is not a win-win situation.

Example 2: Now, in the same town right across the street from the typical cash based clinic, is an insurance-based "Mill Like PT Clinic" that the same patient could also choose.

---

[1] The figures I've picked are a hypothetical numerical value for demonstrating how much benefit is being offered in the marketing message. Therefore, the stronger the marketing message, the higher the perceived benefits, and as such, the higher the figure.

The marketing message of this clinic is "professional, affordable, and a name you can trust". In this case, what they are offering in terms of benefits is actually less than the cash pay clinic (as there's no mention of pain relief, only the safety net of credentials and experience). So, we are going to say that they are only offering 250 units of benefits (significantly less than the cash pay clinic in example 1).

However, and here's where this gets interesting, the cost of care over at the insurance based clinic is just $50 per session (their copay), so the actual value being received by the patient is at 5.

This is higher than the cash pay clinic even though the patient is getting fewer benefits. And, because what the patient really wants is more value, the insurance-based clinic will likely get their business.

AVOID THE RACE TO THE BOTTOM

So what can you learn from this? Well, it is not to drop your rates, a decision which would mean getting into a race to the bottom to see who can provide the most value simply by lowering prices. That is how you go out of business. The only answer is to alter the other element in the equation that you can control - increase the benefits.

Here, I'll show you how to do it with another example:

Example 3: In the same town is a clinic called Paul Gough Physio Rooms (humor me for a moment…). The marketing message, (which includes the **benefit** being promised), at this clinic is "keep active, mobile, free from painkillers, and stay out of the doctor's office – oh, by the way, we'll provide great service, we're all experienced, and we're friendly and qualified as well".

What I have done is something called **"stack the benefits"**. It means the patient sees what they are going to get from hiring me in terms of benefits. You want the patient to see that the benefits are significantly higher than the other two options they have. I am adding 1000 units of benefits to the patient's life – and I'm going to be charging $180 per session to give this to them.

Now according to the value equation, that means the patient will be getting approximately 5.5 units of value from hiring me – even though they are paying me more. I am charging a higher price, but they are hiring me because their **perception** is that they are getting more benefits – so they are still getting more value.

Which, by the way, is what they REALLY wanted in the first place. The cheaper option is just what they felt they had to choose because no other provider gave them a reason not to.

Here's an illustration of how value is increased by "stacking the benefits" in your marketing message – which still lets you charge a higher rate per visit:

FIG.4

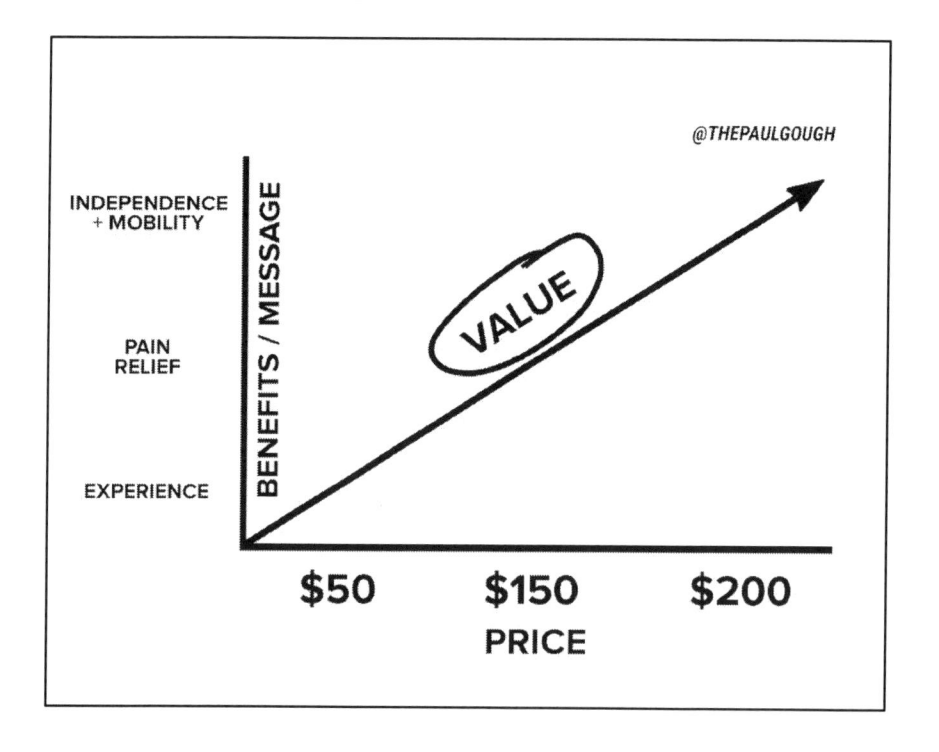

You have heard the saying "show them the value", well this is what that really means. Luckily for me I learned this early on. And instead of spending my whole career trapped inside of the insurance system, always blaming economic conditions in my town, or thinking I could never compete with free socialist medicine, I was able to apply this principle to grow a cash-pay clinic that is able to charge 150% higher prices per session, than the average clinic in England.

The formula that you've just seen is ultimately how I have been able to create a marketing system that let me grow a consistently profitable business. I generate a six figure take home salary for myself despite not being in the treatment room, and barely being in the building anymore (never mind the country!).

Knowing full well that people want more value than saving on their health, I simply jacked up the benefits of what I offer by using my marketing. Did I get more clinically skilled? Of course not. Did I get more experienced? Only one a day at a time. Did I buy new premises or invest in any expensive machines? No. Because none of that is what the patient is interested in. They take all of those things for granted. Patients only care about the **outcome** and what they can do as a result of handing over their time and money. Everything else is simply there to validate a decision already made.

SO HOW DO YOU INCREASE THE PERCEPTION OF BENEFITS?

Here's a key point: value is a concept. Ultimately, value is whatever the person wants it to be, or needs it to be, in order to justify a purchase decision.

Value is not what I want for them, and it is not what you or the profession wants for them. It is only what they want for themselves. And, unbeknownst to most, the value is created at the beginning of their relationship with you and it is based on what they are allowed (by you) to believe they are going to get, which makes the extra investment worthwhile.

And, given that at the beginning they do not know what they are getting until they have paid for it, the only way to be successful is to change their **perception** of what it is that they will be getting from you when they do pay for it.

How do you do that? Easy, you use your marketing, and you constantly fine tune your marketing message so that you resonate with more of the right type of patient - a patient who values what you do enough to want to pay for it.

HERE'S THE NO.1 CASH PAY SUCCESS SECRET

So, you could say that the number one secret to getting more cash pay patients is found by changing the meaning of what your potential patient is going to be paying for.

It is in identifying the target market and tailoring the marketing message to show them how you, **and only you,** know how to provide the benefits they really want (which we discussed this in chapter 1). Do this so clearly that they are happy to pay for it.

Without doing that, you CANNOT make the transition to higher value and much more lucrative, cash paying patients.

In the examples I showed you on the previous pages, easing pain, or restoring function, is a benefit. But it might only carry about 400 units of benefit. If at the Paul Gough Physio Rooms we are solving a patient's lack of mobility, helping someone maintain independence, helping her avoid surgery, or we're helping to stop her liver from "rotting" as a result of a dependence on pain medication, then the numerical value placed against the benefits we are providing is obviously significantly higher, in fact, much closer to 1000.

I am offering a lot more (as they see it), so I am able to charge more and they are happy to pay for it. It is only in the marketing message that the difference is found. You might be providing the same type of service, but patients have to believe before hiring you that it is going to be more tailored to them, and that it will provide the **outcome** that they want.

You might be less qualified or less experienced, but if you are talking about outcomes and benefits, and your competition is talking credentials and qualifications, you will win. I am living proof of this, and I have hundreds of case studies from clinic owners from all over the world who have used this formula to back it up (many featured at the front of this book and some fresh out of school).

USE YOUR MARKETING TO PROMISE A COMPLETELY DIFFERENT OUTCOME

I keep saying it, but I don't think I can stress this point enough - using your marketing to promise an outcome that is unachievable anywhere else is the ONLY way to win.

The core of any business success is the **PROMISE** made to the customer about the outcome that will be delivered (not how skilled the person who providing it is). Only when that is established do the patients start to care about credentials and experience, not before.

If you cannot use your marketing to establish the value that they will receive, then they will never get to the point of caring about credentials or experience. The patient simply will not pay the difference. Patients will always choose the cheaper option, and you will always find yourself blaming the situation, your town's economy, or whatever else struggling business owners like to blame for their predicament.

Here it is in a very blunt summary: the difference between whether or not people will pay in cash (or not at all) is found in what you let them believe the outcome they will get from you is. If your focus is "intrinsic", i.e. on your clinical skills, then they **will not pay** the difference you are asking.

However, if your focus is on them, and you use your marketing to clearly show that you are focused on their specific pain points, showing how you can solve them better than anyone else, then **they will pay** the difference. That is it.

It does not require more clinical skills, only better **marketing skills.**

With all of that said, let me give you a few specific examples of what I mean by "change the meaning". I'll show you how you might do it in your marketing to make attracting cash pay patients much easier:

"CHANGE THE MEANING – CHANGE THE OUTCOME"

In a marketing situation you might run an ad in the local newspaper or on Facebook, announcing that you are the most professional or most qualified physical therapist in town, with the promise to fix pain or restore function.

The "meaning" – the thing that the customer believes you stand for – is now a physical therapist who provides pain relief or restores function. Suppose you run a small ad to begin with and you don't get as many calls as you would like, but you are certain that the ad looks good and the right people are reading the newspaper, so you decide to run a bigger version of the same ad. What then? Nothing changes except the ad is now twice the size (and twice the price).

The meaning of the services being offered has not changed, and so the result remains the same - not as many calls as you hoped for, not even enough to make the ad worth running despite the increased visibility. So the solution is to change what the ad means to the person who is seeing it.

For example: instead of your ad being all about physical therapy, the ad needs to be about something that actually matters to the patient - their independence, getting back into the CrossFit box, being able to walk for a period of time without needing to dash to the toilet, or going surfing on their own (because they can put their own clothing on independently) – in other words, all of the things that having less pain and more function would allow them to finally do. If you change the meaning of what you do for patients, you nearly always change the outcome.

Now what's funny is that when I first started to teach this principle, physical therapists would tell me "but it's obvious that is what I meant", or, "that's what I would help them to achieve if they came to see me". And my response is always the same, "if they have to think about the meaning of your services, they won't – and your marketing will fail."

Here's an example of what I mean by that last statement. It's a very famous marketing experiment carried out on a blind man who was begging for money…

"I'M BLIND… PLEASE HELP!"

Picture the scene: there's a blind man sitting slouched against a wall. He's wearing scruffy clothes, is unshaven, and looks like he hasn't had a bath for a month. He's got his plastic bags next to him, which contain everything that he owns, and at the other side of him is a hat for people to drop money in to help him out. What is also next to him is a piece of cardboard with the words "I'm blind, please help" written in big block capital letters, easily visible to anyone who walks by. And there are 1000's walking by.

He is positioned in such a great spot that it is hard not to see him and his sign. In four hours thousands of people walk right past him and, in total, he is given just a few measly dollars. Very few people leave the guy any money despite his request for "help" even though he is blind and obviously unable to fend for himself.

What happens next is astounding and could be one of the **most important marketing lessons I've ever learned.** While the guy sits and continues to beg, a woman walks up to him and picks up his sign, turns it over, and writes something on it. The lady puts the sign back down (the blind man is oblivious to it) and she walks away to watch and record what happens.

What happens next? Well, $100's get dropped into the same hat that had been empty all morning. Nothing else changed. The same guy was still in the same spot just as blind. There were the same number of people walking by him as there was earlier in the day. So what was the new message on the sign?

It changed from "I'm blind, please help", to "it's a beautiful day outside and I won't see any of it". Same thing – different meaning, and as a result there was a completely different outcome.

YOUR PATIENTS DO THIS AS WELL

The human brain is very lazy and does not want to have to convert things like "I'm blind please help" to what that really means, which is – that the guy begging will never get to see the same beautiful day that we, with our eyesight intact, can.

It wasn't that people didn't have the money to give him, they just couldn't find the motivation to do it and they know what they were doing it for. Common sense tells you that we would all understand the implications of being blind, namely that he wouldn't see the beautiful day. But, there's a big difference between common sense and common practice, and the result of our behavior is actually different depending on the angle.

How many thousands of physical therapists around the world today are scratching their heads wondering why, despite needing their services, people in pain with "functional problems", will not see the value in their great service? It is because the exact same thing is going on here. They can't see it. They don't understand the meaning of it clearly.

They can't conclude for themselves that an end to pain and functional issues will lead them to being able to do the things they really want. So it is your job to spell it out to them in both your marketing and your internal communication. It is your job to change the sign from "we ease your pain", to, "we help you keep your independence". If you do that you'll end up with a hat full of dollars from people wanting to do business with you, all because you made it easy for them to connect the meaning of your service with the outcome they really want.

(*The actual video of this marketing experiment is included in your book purchase bonus pack for you to watch. You can get it by going to www.paulgough.com/resource)

LESSONS FROM WALT DISNEY ON HOW TO MARKET YOUR CLINIC

Changing the meaning of your services in the manner I am showing you now not only changes the volume of response you get, it also changes the quality of the calls you get. Like I said earlier, we do not want more patients for more patients sake – we want more PROFIT, and one of the many things that directly affect the volume and quality of leads that you get is your "marketing message", which clearly states the outcome that you are promising.

Your marketing message is your way of communicating precisely what it is that you want your potential patients to believe: what you stand for and will do for them. As you now know, this directly impacts what you can charge and what they will be happy to pay for.

It is your way of demonstrating that you understand the ultimate outcome wanted, the one that the patient believes she will get if she agrees to hire you. Here's the thing: you have to think very carefully about what it is that you want to be known for. Similarly, if Disney was defined by "roller coasters" and "rides" in its theme parks, they wouldn't be making that much money, and neither will you if all you stand for is being the most professional and friendly physical therapist in town.

Let me explain: at Disney, instead of just getting on a roller coaster, you are going to go on a "journey through space". Walt Disney realized from the get-go that people would not stand in line for 90 minutes (in the 100-degree heat and humidity of Orlando) just for a roller coaster. But he knew that they would do it for the promise of a "magical journey through space".

If Disney's marketing message had been about a theme park with great roller coasters, even a place where you can have a lot of fun, it wouldn't be as popular as it is today. What is more, he would have gotten a theme park full of people all moaning about the length of the queues, the temperature, and the ridiculously short ride times. He would have spent about ten years asking himself why everyone who comes to the theme park doesn't seem to want to spend any money and never wants to come back. He would have either gone broke, or given up. Either way, he would not have been left with the same "rides" and the same "theme park" that Disney currently has today. The exact same theme parks that are currently making billions of dollars each year.

The point I am making is this - nothing but the right marketing message separates Disney from all of the other cheaper options that try and struggle to make a theme park work on a large scale.

At Disney you are going to the "Happiest Place on Earth". You're going to make memories with your family that last a lifetime, and, you are happy to pay way more than any other "theme park" for it. You do crazy things like spend twice as much as you budgeted for and you leave happy that you did. Often you're so happy that you'll rush back next year (and every year after that if possible) to do it all again.

I've been going to Disney with my family for 25 years, and in that time the "big three" rollercoasters at *Magic Kingdom* – 'Space Mountain', 'Thunder Mountain', and 'Splash Mountain' – have not changed or improved once. What has changed? The price to ride the things! The cost of admission to ride an out of date rollercoaster has gone up significantly, and it is making Disney a very profitable company.

Imagine if a new theme park tried to add a ride that was built in the 70's, and not only that, it charged you $100 per day to ride it? I don't think they'd last very long, do you? It is Disney's marketing message that makes it possible for them to charge so much. The distinction here is profound and shouldn't be lost on you.

If you're not getting the type of response from your marketing that you want, or you're not getting the "types" of patients that you want (i.e. those happy to pay in cash), then it is because you are allowing them to think what you are offering is a "roller coaster" when in fact, what they want is a "journey through space". It is because your marketing message is off point. What's more, if your staff are talking gleefully about all the benefits of physical therapy, then basically all you're saying is how great the car is that you'll sit in when the roller coaster ride starts. Who cares how great the car is? Tell me all about the thrills that I'll get when I go through "space" at 60 mph screaming endlessly with excitement at the same time as my family, or when I leave having created memories and stories of the journey that will last a lifetime (and a picture that I can buy for $15 to take home with me).

Those are the benefits that the customer wants and why Disney is able to charge more, (and has more repeat customers), than any other theme park. Remember, **Value = Benefits / Price**. Disney racks up the benefits before you have even arrived. They do that by changing the perception of what it is that you will find there. It's very often the case that what you are looking for, you find.

I took this lesson from Walt Disney; at the Paul Gough Physio Rooms a life without pills, one with more independence, with more sustained activity, and one with an increase in mobility, is the equivalent of the "journey through space". It is what separates me from all of my competitors, and you need to find your equivalent if your marketing is to be more successful (I'll show you how to do it in chapter 6 and 7).

PEOPLE PAY MORE FOR SOLUTIONS TO INTERNAL PROBLEMS

As I said from the outset of this chapter, marketing success is about the **PROMISE** that you make to solve the patient's specific problems. The bigger the promise, the more marketing success. The bigger the difference you can promise to make (and ethically back up), the more success you will have. Given that marketing is really about how much, and how well you can motivate someone to do something (like call you or arrive at your clinic), then ultimately, the success of your clinics marketing will stand and fall on the ability of your marketing system. Your system needs to motivate someone enough to get in touch with you. How well you can motivate the patient to want to have their problem solved by you, and only you, is something you have to consider. I've learned that the best and most impactful way to motivate someone is to promise to solve their internal problems, not just their external ones.

This is another subtle difference between a marketing campaign that does not fail and one that does, and your understanding of this is **vital** to your marketing success.

Whenever you see world-class companies, they usually have world-class marketing. You rarely get one without the other, and what these world-class companies have in common is that they immediately focus their marketing on showing the potential customer what **internal problem** the product or service solves.

For example, Apple shows you how their 'iPad' connects you to your children via the pictures you can take on it, or family movies you can effortlessly make using it. On the other hand, Samsung shows you how fast their latest processer is.

Now, don't get me wrong, I am not suggesting that Samsung is not a successful company. I am however suggesting there's a reason why Apple has more money in the bank than any other company in the world, and it is unlikely to be because their processor is superior. After all, what customer would ever know the difference anyway? Like Disney, all of their marketing is about providing a solution to an internal problem.

In our world, whatever "pain" or loss of function that your prospective patient has, it is making them feel a certain way. That could be "worried", "frustrated", "frightened", "insecure", "skeptical" or "nervous".

I've learned, through $100,000's spent on marketing, that until you solve that problem, you'll never get the chance to solve the external problem. To take this one step further, I actually use the words 'frustrated', 'worried', 'nervous' etc., in my clinic's marketing. I talk to the patients directly about how they are feeling internally, and then I link it directly to the external problem they're living with.

An example might be this: "Are you <u>worried</u> about losing your ability to walk in the hands of knee pain?" Notice how I lead with the internal problem whilst at the same time I acknowledge the external problem (their knee pain). Understanding this not only changed the level of response I got from my marketing, but also changed the relationship I was having with those who responded all for the better.

Patients who see and respond to marketing that focuses on solving their internal problems come to you much more committed, more open to asking for your help, more trusting of your diagnosis, and deeply committed to believing in your plan of care (they are also happy to pay in cash!). If that is what you want, then you will only get that result by talking to them about their internal problems. This can only be done through the use of marketing and a continuation of building trust in the early stages of the relationship, i.e. when they first make contact with your clinic. I'll show you exactly how to do it in chapters 6, 7 and 8.

5

FINDING THE FORTUNE ALREADY IN YOUR CLINIC

The number one most overlooked aspect of any clinic's marketing is the "follow up" process. If you are hearing the term "follow up" for the first time, then it's likely that it's missing from your clinic. And that's exactly why it is important that we cover it today. You need to understand why you need it.

"Follow up" is not something that is optional. It is the critical missing link between doing "ok" in your marketing, and making a fortune in your marketing. It is the difference between an inquiry and a paying patient. It is the difference between "what's the price?" And an actual scheduled evaluation with you. It is the difference between "I am just calling to find out how physical therapy works", and then an actual plan of care being implemented and completed.

Here's the point: most people think that marketing is just about getting the phone to ring, but it is much more about what you do **after** the phone rings that will determine the ROI you will get from your marketing. Having a follow up system changed everything for me, and I can quite openly tell you that at least 50% of the people who do business with me today originally said "no", "I'll think about it", or the classic, "I'll get back to you". Yet, they eventually agreed to be a patient, and that is all because of my follow up system.

It is only because of this follow up system, or 'Attraction System' (discussed in chapter 7), that I am able to turn a "no" into a "yes". That I am able to change an "I'll get back to you", into an "I'll see you Tuesday at 3pm, Paul". As a result, I am much more profitable *and* I now need less leads. That's a win-win.

"$1,000,000 LOST BY NOT HAVING A FOLLOW UP SYSTEM"

True story: I coined the phrase "the fortune is in the follow up" during a coaching call with a client of mine, namely, Dean Volk (of *Volk PT* in North and South Carolina). At that time, I pointed out to him that one of the most overlooked ways of adding profit to a business is to "follow up" with all of the people who ever made an inquiry at your clinic, even if they had started and later dropped off, or even worse, just didn't show up when they said they would.

Wherever you are on your business journey, as you read this book remember that this principle applies to you, and that it will either make you money if you adhere to it, or will cost you money if you choose to ignore it. Now, in the case of the Dean, he is an established business owner with a 10+ years history of running a business. When we first met, he asked me about the fastest ways to become more profitable. It was then I asked him to do a calculation. I asked him to calculate the total number of people who had called his office, not scheduled, had scheduled but failed to arrive, or had started but dropped off later on. He spent 60 seconds or so scribbling down a rough estimate of the number. It was well over 100. I then asked him to remind me of how much the typical patient was worth to his business. He said $1200. I didn't need a calculator to conclude that he was losing a small fortune in not having a process in play that, basically, factors in the principles discussed in chapter 1 (that people in Group 2 are not always ready to "book now", in spite of making inquiries that suggest they might be).

We continued to talk and after a while we got a little more granular and worked out a figure: 100 patients (not followed up on) X $1200 average value = $120,000. **That is a lot of money.** It makes my stomach sick just thinking about the fact that Dean had technically lost it. But now, factor in that this has been going on for 10 years or more. Astonishingly, we're now at over $1,000,000 in money that has, quite literally, walked out of his clinic. That is 1 million dollars that could have been his if only it had been followed up on. Now I don't feel sick anymore. I feel faint. I am about to keel over for him.

Take a moment to calculate that number for your practice, using the last year as a time scale. Insert the numbers as appropriate:

_____ Number of people who have called the office and didn't schedule.

_____ Number of people who have scheduled an appointment, but didn't show up.

_____ Number of people who started treatment, but didn't complete.

Now take the total of the above 3 numbers = _____
Multiply that by the avg. patient value/spend = _____ 1 year lost revenue.

Multiply the 1 year lost revenue X _____ of years in practice.

_____ Total amount lost since opening by not having a follow up system.

"ENOUGH TO PAY FOR A HOLIDAY HOME IN CHARLESTON!"

Granted, you wouldn't get all of this $1,000,000 coming to you, not even with the best follow up system in the world. But even with the worst follow up system you would still get about 30% of it. Because all that is needed for 1 in 3 of these people who drop off, don't show, or just fail to carry on with their inquiry, is a simple system to nurture and/or reactivate them. Dean and I continued the conversation and agreed that if just 30% of the patients in his 10 years of running a business (who were allowed to walk out the door) were put back on schedule, then his net-worth would look very different than it does today. "How different?" I asked him. He said, and I quote, "I'd have enough to pay off my house in Charleston!" And that is precisely why I say, "the Fortune is in the Follow Up". Because it is. And to make your marketing work, you are going to need to have a follow up system in place (we will create this for you in chapter 8).

If you are an established business, save yourself the agony of looking back at how much not having a follow up system has cost you (and immediately follow the steps I'll teach you in chapter 8). And, if you are a new business owner, congratulations! I've just given you a clear path to owning a second home in Charleston, debt free, within 10 years. (You are welcome!)

YOU CANNOT GROW A BUSINESS WITHOUT LEAD GENERATION

For all the reasons mentioned in chapter 1, you cannot grow a business without predictable lead generation. And you cannot make lead generation work without a follow up system that takes your potential patient on a journey that leads to him to making a decision to buy from you. Lead generation marketing is about attracting qualified leads. It is not about asking people to book now. It is about starting a relationship with someone who has a problem you can solve, and it's about educating them on how you can help them solve their problem.

The follow up system is about guiding the potential patient along a series of steps so that they become ready to buy. Remember, we are marketing to the people in **Group 2**, those we identified in chapter 1; those who need what you do, but are just not quite ready to buy from you (yet!). This is the target market with the overwhelming majority, and focusing on this group is the only chance you have of being successful with your marketing. For that reason and more, you need a follow up system.

The follow up system bridges the gap between what they know now and what they need to know to confidently book and pay for your services.

INVALUABLE INSIGHTS ABOUT YOUR PATIENTS

A great marketing system not only provides you with quality leads to help you grow your practice predictably, it also gives you amazing insights into your patients and their decision making. And that is going to help you no-end when it comes to improving conversion and compliance. The more you know and understand your patients, as well as how they make their decisions, the more you are able to help them. And over the years since doing all of this, I have learned more than I could have ever imagined about how patients think and act.

For example, the biggest thing that I've learned is that the odds of them saying NO to your services are significantly higher than the odds of them saying "yes". Of course, we are going to put a follow up system in place in your business to reverse this, but to give you the best shot at being truly successful with regards to helping your patients make better decisions about hiring you, it's going to help you tremendously if you first understand all of the major forces that are in play causing people to say NO.

This will not only help in your clinic's marketing, your internal communication will improve too. Additionally, when it comes to converting patients to a full plan of care, talking about prices, and even stopping things like drop offs, no-shows, and cancellations, things will also improve. So, with that in mind, let me share some of the things that I've learned about why "no one wants to pay for your services" and what to do about it.

WHY NO ONE WANTS TO PAY FOR YOUR SERVICES – AND WHAT YOU CAN DO ABOUT IT

With the cost of health care rising, the "price" is likely to be the number one reason why people object. No doubt you hear, "I can't afford it", or "it's too expensive" every day. I do too. But here's the thing - if they say "no" at hearing your fees it is often not that they don't have the money, or that they do not want to pay what you ask, it is simply that they are not able to say yes right away. **Human beings are not hard wired to be able to make impulse decisions on anything over $100.**

That means if I see something under $100 – an item of clothing for example – even though I wasn't planning on buying it that day, there's a high chance I will buy it anyway (assuming I like it).

It is an impulse decision.

But, as soon as the price rises above $100 it is common for us to want to delay the decision, and it then becomes what is called a "destination" decision. That means the customer will deliberate over it for a few days or weeks (maybe longer), and then, when they have decided they are happy to pay for it, that is if they conclude the value is there, they will go to the most appropriate destination to get the item they have decided to buy. The difference between not buying and buying is simply **'time'**.

Essentially, when something is over $100 we put thought into buying it to ensure we get the decision right. Or to be more scientific, to make sure we don't get it wrong! This type of purchasing decision is happening in your life (and mine) every day, from how you choose your vacations or the restaurants you dine in, to gifts you buy for your kids. You and your patients are no different.

Here's an example: my favorite toy store is Geppetto's in La Jolla, San Diego. I go there regularly with my son Harry. He might for example, see a water gun that he wants to play with in our pool. He will bring it over to show me, suggesting that I might buy it for him. When he does this, my first instinct is to look for the little sticker on the back to check the price. I am instinctively looking to see if it is below $100. If it is priced at, say, $27.99, I will tell him to put it in the shopping basket (and hope that his mother doesn't notice when we get to the checkout!). However, if it is $127.99 there are now three digits before the dot, and my reaction is likely to be something completely different altogether.

"Ask your Grandmother"... is the usual line I use if it's above $100!

Because it is over $100 I am not going to make a snap purchase decision, I will be absolving myself from having to make that decision by making that statement. Instead, I suggest that it might be something that his Grandmother might like to buy him for his birthday or Christmas. I'm delaying the decision making process to make sure there are no consequences of getting it wrong. My capacity threshold for making quick decisions is set at $100.

It is the same with restaurants. If it is a regular Friday evening and Natalie and I want to eat out, we might choose to go to somewhere like TGI Fridays. That is an easy decision to make. Why? Because I know that the bill will be less than $100. However, going to somewhere like Morton's or Fleming's steakhouse on a Friday night would have to be planned months in advance. The reality of frequenting those types of restaurants is they need to be justified by a birthday, or a special occasion, like when family come into town. That's because I know the total bill at these places will be well over $100.

SCHOOLED BY AN "OUT OF DATE" SYSTEM

So, how is this relevant to you? Well, you've likely been schooled by a system that has taught you how to interact with patients in a scenario where the total cost of physical therapy was likely to be less than $100. The average copay was likely to be around $10 per session. And, if the prescription of care was for 10 visits, the total cost of physical therapy owed by the patient was coming in at $100. No problem – it is an impulse decision that patients can easily commit to.

It is deciding to go to TGI Fridays or to buy the smaller water pistol for my son, Harry. Fast forward to today and what is the total cost of physical therapy? For some, their copay contribution for one session alone could be $100! The average insurance patient is facing a bill of up to $50 per session for their copay, and if the clinic is suggesting 10 sessions, then the total bill is going to be closer to $500. The typical insurance clinic has moved from TGI Fridays to Morton's. From the "water pistol", to the "super soaker", and if I am a patient in your clinic, I am now seriously considering whether or not I go any further with you.

It is not that I don't want to, it is just my natural instinct to want to take time to decide whether or not there is value in it for me. And even then, it is a knee-jerk reaction to deliberate whether or not I should just wait a couple of months to see if this back pain eases on its own.

THIS IS ONLY GOING TO GET WORSE

Now, the reality is that the price that they will need to pay you, or I, is not going to go down any time soon. So, this resistance, this pushback, this not wanting to pay or comply issue (that so many clinics are facing right now), is not only blindingly obvious – it is going to get worse. If you are a cash-pay clinic, you are the equivalent of a Morton's steakhouse. You are the super soaker. You are now a destination purchase and your patient is going to need time.

You are not an impulse purchase, and all of this has to be factored in to the way you market your clinic, how you talk to patients, and the system you use. Fail to address it and my guess is you will get stuck where you are.

The solution is to factor in that people need time to deliberate over you and the value you are proposing to bring to their lives. If they tell you "no", it does not mean that they are saying, "no, I don't want you", it just means that they are saying "no, not right now". There's a difference. It means they need time and more information, and that means you need a system in your business which delivers the information to bridge the gap. Having a system also ensures that the patient who says "no, not right now" does not get forgotten, or possibly be assumed to be the wrong type of patient.

I put it to you that this "I'm not sure" behavior is perfectly normal, and if you pay attention to this advice and you create a follow up system in your business, then this will be the difference (that makes the difference) to your profits. **It is that important.** Keep this in mind: just because they said "no", or "I'll need to think about it", does not mean that they don't want you – it just means that they need to "ask Grandma!"

YOUR PATIENTS ARE NOT VERY GOOD AT MAKING DECISIONS

Another reason why your marketing needs a follow up system is that, as humans, we are not hardwired to be comfortable with making decisions. Most people would rather accept unhappiness over risking uncertainty, and for that reason alone they find it difficult to make decisions. Hiring a physical therapist in their world can seem like a very risky decision. The cost, the possibility of taking their clothes off, the pain afterwards, and the risk of the issue not actually getting any better (despite spending money), all make it difficult for them to make the decision and say yes.

And that's a problem for us. Because for any commercial transaction to happen, (between a customer and business), the customer has to make a decision. In our world, the patient has to make a commitment to you. They have to make three commitments – with their time, their money, and their trust. That is hard for them to do.

The fallacy in a business like ours is that just because the patients are in pain, all of their natural tendencies towards indecisiveness are forgotten and they will just pick up the phone and sort it out. After all – they are in pain. But that is not how it works.

In the absence of a referral from a doctor they are incredibly indecisive, not to mention skeptical. So, if you are trying to make direct to consumer marketing work, your entire marketing system has to be designed to factor in that almost everyone you will come into contact with will struggle to make a decision to say yes.

It doesn't mean that they won't say yes, it just means you have to focus your attention on the fact that it is a struggle for them – a natural struggle – and you will be rewarded for helping them to make a decision.

Simply being aware of this is likely to bring you more success, and sadly, most business owners spend their whole careers oblivious of this fact. Instead, they assume that anyone who stalls or is indecisive is a time waster, doesn't want to pay, or is not the right patient. It is arrogant and ignorant to assume that. It's much better to take the position that **you** just haven't done enough to help them reach a decision yet.

The former is a world that is full of frustration. The latter is significantly more profitable, I assure you.

Here's something else: when the patients are in pain, or thinking negatively about their future, they are even less likely to make a good decision. As the saying goes, "confused buyers buy nothing", and this ultimately means that patients (much like Mary and Christine who I introduced you to in chapter 1) will deliberate more and more. The only decision that they are ever going to make is that they need to think about it even more. Their decision is that they can't decide, so they tell you they need more time (and so this goes on, and on, sometimes for years).

You could say that a huge part of my clinic's success has been because I have truly immersed myself in accepting this principle as fact. I have built my entire marketing system and business around understanding this one principle about human behavior - and it has been liberating. There's no more frustration when a patient makes an inquiry and doesn't go ahead – I accept that they just needed more time. There's no more getting anxious at wondering why patients who called my office to request free information didn't call us back for three months. The reality is that they hadn't even considered me an option before seeing the ad (and therefore needed to feel more comfortable before taking the next step). I accepted that it was my job to create the right system to make them feel more comfortable, and having the follow up system makes that happen effortlessly.

Since understanding this there's no more making rash decisions about "marketing not working" if a patient didn't book right there and then. The reality is that I just had false expectations about how fast I thought the marketing would work. Educating myself about both marketing, and the people I am marketing to, allowed me to change my understanding of the situation, and as a consequence, get very different results.

I've learned that the reality is very few people are ever ready to hand over money to you right off the bat. This is true for any profession or industry. I am not that special to be an exception to the rule. The problem for many physical therapists is, as I see it, that they are so used to doctors spoon-feeding them patients who are "ready to buy now" (Group 3), that this world of having to nurture and guide people on a journey to make a decision is not only alien, it is frustrating.

I believe some physical therapists will even think it is beneath them. It is as if the resume should sell itself. Bad news – it doesn't.

A lot of people in this profession have had it lucky for a long, long time. They have literally been "spoon-fed" their customers from one referral source for so long.

Of course, that referral source was the doctor. That meant no one ever had to learn how to nurture a relationship with a real customer (only the doctor). No one had to learn any of this before now, and in the past it was just a case of call and see the doctor every Monday, drop off the cookies and lunches for the staff, and wait for the referrals to flood in.

The reality is, that isn't the case anymore. Those referrals from doctors dry up, and clinic owners are now finding out that in the "real world" of direct real marketing it is not as simple as a patient arriving with a script in one hand and an insurance card in the other. It is very seldom that a patient is ready to buy a ten session plan of care.

This idea that customers will somehow just show up and hand over money is madness to most successful business owners. And that is precisely why they are successful; they are able to embrace the idea that customers are skeptical and indecisive by design, and win anyway.

PHYSICAL THERAPY IS A GRUDGE PURCHASE

Another reason that you need a follow up system in your clinic is that people do not value their health as much as they would have you believe, or as much as you've been led to believe. There are no lectures at PT school that teach you the difference between 'saying' and 'doing'. This concept can be confusing for a private practice owner who assumes that he is in a profession that provides the type of service everyone needs.

For example: ask people if they value their health and of course they'll tell you they do. However, the reality of the decisions we make regarding things like food, activity, and fitness (the stuff that affects our health), will often tell a different story. Ask a guy 200lb overweight if he values his health and he'll tell you he does. He'll believe it too. But his actions are telling you that, in principle, he values it yes, but when it comes to actually doing something about it, it's a very different story.

I think what people are often trying to say is that they WANT to value their health – they just don't know how to do it. And the fact that people do not value their health as much as they think they do is not a great starting point when trying to build a private pay clinic. If you are not careful, you can easily be "duped" into thinking that everyone is going to want to do something about ill health. You might even believe that running a health business is going to be easy because, surely, anyone with ill health will want to restore it. They don't.

And when you think about it (unemotionally) no one really wants to spend money with us. We are not a sexy or exciting service. Sure, we provide a great service to people, but it is hardly something that people approach with a spring in their step, feeling excited about having to do. And besides, they're used to being able to go to bed and waking up with their problem gone.

WHY 50 IS THE MAGIC NUMBER

The problem that we have and why so many stall over coming to see us, is that it is not until the age of about 50 that people actually start valuing their health enough to want to pay for it.

Sadly, this narrows down the target market to about one third of the population. 50 is pivotal, because at that point things start to go wrong, or the patient takes a lot longer to recover. It is at this point in their lives that people finally start to face up to the fact that they are losing a grip on their independence and mobility, and only then are they more inclined to want to do something to protect or restore it.

Loss, or the fear of loss, is one of the most powerful motivators in life. If your ideal patient is below 50, this might explain why it is difficult to get them to say yes to the plan of care that they really need; the plan of care that is perfect for them to help them achieve their said goal. This is the same plan of care that they just do not seem to want to pay for, no matter what you say.

Having a follow up system helps you, because what starts as "I'll see how it goes" oftentimes ends up being accepted as the "this is how it has to be". This results in you being forgotten about. If a patient doesn't instantly see the value in paying for what you are offering, then a follow up system is your way of staying in touch with them until they do see the value.

Often times, the only difference between a patient who does not immediately see the value and then later does, is time - a few more frustrated months not being able to do what it is that they want to do. You just have to make sure that you are visible when this frustration hits boiling point.

If you can do that, and you can be there at their boiling point, it is my experience that you will inherit a significantly different patient – one who now views you very favorably, and is willing to listen to what you have to say and what you propose to do for them.

WHAT GETS DONE ANYTIME - GETS DONE NO TIME

The case for the inclusion of a follow up system which is bolted onto your marketing, is never ending. Here's another reason why it is needed, and why growing a physical therapy clinic can prove so challenging for so many… There's a great saying that pretty much sums up how most of us live our lives, "if it can get done anytime – it usually gets done no time".

Typically as physical therapists we are not in the "life and death" business. We are in the business of improving quality of life. And people can improve that "anytime" they like. Which is why we are often second, third, fourth or even fifth on the list of priorities of the things that people choose to do before they get to us. Think about booking a flight somewhere: how many times have you promised yourself that "tonight is the night that you are going to go online and book it", yet you never actually get round to booking it. And when you eventually do book that flight, the price is 5x than what it would have been had you done it weeks ago.

I do the same thing all the time. Patients do it too. If they can call anytime, they are likely to do it in "no time".

Having a system in place makes it significantly more likely that "today" will be the day that they do call you. With your emails, your calls, your direct mail (all of the things that go into a follow up system), you are able to give them a valid reason to call – today. You are able to get to the top of the priority list because you can stress the urgency of what it is they need to do; in this way they can't possibly risk putting you off for yet another day.

I am sure you have heard it from your patients - "I've been meaning to call you... I just never got round to it". I used to hear it all the time from patients telling me that they just kept forgetting to call me. If it is happening to you, then there are appointments not being booked in your schedule that should be. It is costing you a small fortune and the patient is in a lot more pain, and experiencing a lot more stiffness, than he needs to be living with.

THERE'S NO INSTANT GRATIFICATION WITH PHYSICAL THERAPY

One more reason why "no-one wants to pay for physical therapy" is that what we do takes some time to yield an outcome. That is known as "delayed gratification", and what people are being conditioned to want right now is "instant gratification".

We offer delayed gratification at a premium – what patients want is instant gratification at cheaper, half price, or with a discount thrown in for good measure. We are a profession that is going in the opposite direction to what people are wanting to buy these days, and that is creating a bigger problem for us as our costs rise.

When people contemplate booking an appointment with us they are aware it could take weeks, or even months, to get their desired outcome. And that is a problem. There isn't a part of their brain that makes them suddenly happy to want to wait for their benefits after handing over thousands of dollars or more for their product or service. I've said it many times, there are no "bags of stuff" in the business we're in. There is just a "promise" of an outcome we have to hope the patient believes will be delivered. It is blind-faith in you and I, someone that they have never met and don't know much about, that needs to prevail.

Contrast that with buying something like a TV off Amazon (where your new TV is up on the wall and you're watching Netflix within 24 hours). Think of going to Walmart and spending $100 – you walk out with bags of "stuff" to load into the trunk of the car and eat within minutes of driving off. There's some understanding and justification in handing over your money: you got something tangible.

Instant gratification does not happen with us, and that is going to be an ever-increasing problem as it gets more expensive. Using your marketing correctly (like I showed you in chapter 3), and continuing to communicate with patients using a follow up system, helps the patients see more clearly what it is they are actually buying. It helps patients justify the purchase and understand why the benefits haven't arrived as quickly as when they go to the dentist or even their hairdresser.

Very few sciatica problems are fixed in 60 minutes. Very few hamstring strains are solved in one visit. Very few mechanical lower back problems are sorted (properly) in one session. Now sure, your patients are going to get "some relief" when they first come in, but they also know that there's going to be a lot more to do after that first visit. That though for many is enough to keep them from ever starting.

This is "lack of instant gratification" is a problem you and I face, and it is rarely ever discussed. And that is precisely why it is a problem. Everything that I've discussed in this chapter (and more) is what you are up against everyday as you battle for customers' hearts, minds, and ultimately, their wallets, purses, or insurance cards. The more you are aware of the real problem that is holding the patients back, and you're not constantly blaming the "system", "your town", or "marketing not working for health care", the more likely you are to be successful in business.

The goal of this chapter was to bring these roadblocks to your attention so that they are much easier to spot and navigate. We all have a blind spot – a scotoma - and for many physical therapists that blind spot is often tunnel vision. It only sees everything good about the profession we love, it is not able to accept or see the reasons why people might not be quite as "in love" with it as we are.

It is when you are able to take the stance of the latter that there are more reasons that they might not book than reasons they should book, that more marketing success will come your way. This is why I wanted to include just some of them in this book.

THERE'S MORE ON THE PODCAST

If you want to find out more about "why people do not always want to pay for physical therapy", I spoke in-depth about many of these key principles (and more) in a keynote presentation that I was invited to give at the American Physical Therapy Association (APTA) Private Practice Section (PPS) Annual Conference in Chicago, 2017. Over 10,000 private practice owners attended the same event and the entire talk is available to download and listen to on my **Physical Therapy Business School Podcast:** www.paulgough.com/podcast/audio-experience-35

After you have finished reading this book, I invite you to go the podcast and listen to me speak about these principles as well. I am sure you will pick up something new or possibly even hear something in a way not covered in this book.

6

3 STEPS TO GROW YOUR PRACTICE PROFITS USING MARKETING THAT ACTUALLY WORKS

Marketing done right, "Paul Style", is fundamentally about building relationships, trust, and confidence in you, the outcome, and in the patient themselves. If all you are selling is your credentials and experience, then you are asking them to make a huge commitment with you before any of that is achieved. Selling appointments right off the bat is hard at the best of times and it is almost impossible if it is not backed up by a strong marketing message.

With that in mind, let's look more specifically at what you need to do to make the lead generation and relationship marketing strategy work for you at your clinic.

STEP #1: PICK YOUR PERFECT PATIENT (TARGET MARKET)

Earlier on in the book I raised the idea that you need to get clear on a specific target market in order to run your ads effectively. Well, now it's time to decide who that is going to be.

Selecting an "ideal" or "perfect" patient is vital, because it forces you to think long and hard about the problems that she is living with. It also gives your marketing the ability to show how you can solve those problems better than anyone else. That is your unique serving proposition. That, and that alone, is what is going to make you different from your competition. After all, soon every physical therapist will be a "doctor", and if everyone one has the same 'D' before their name, at what point does that make you a commodity?...

GENERALISTS GO BROKE - SPECIALISTS GET RICH!

One of the reasons that physical therapists struggle to charge higher prices than say personal trainers, (or even hairdressers in some instances), is because we graduate as **generalists.** We have been taught to do a "little bit of everything", and as a result, never really specialize in anything. And that is a problem, because specialists are who people seek and ultimately, spend the most money with. Generalists try to help everyone - and get tired and go broke.

Specialists narrow down to a specific target market, they charge more money to provide that specialist service, and as a result, they get rich! What do you want to spend your career doing?

When you get clear on your ideal patient you start the process of becoming a specialist, and because you can start to talk about their specific problems, in the eyes of that perfect patient you are becoming "everything" (rather than a little bit of something to everyone).

At first, it might seem counter-intuitive that you are going to choose to ignore some people and instead focus on a small pocket of people, but what needs to be understood is that if people can't find themselves in the ad or the marketing message you are putting out, they will ignore it. And that's a problem, because without getting their attention they are not going to take action, and if they don't take action they will not come and see you.

Sure, there might be 5000 people seeing your ad on *Facebook*, but if it isn't talking to someone with a specific problem, and isn't showing how you can solve it, then no one is noticing it.

"WHO PAYS YOU THE MOST MONEY WITHOUT ANY QUESTIONS ASKED?"

If you are "stuck" or are finding it difficult to select your perfect patient, just ask yourself this question: "Who pays you the most money with the least amount of hassle?" Now think about how much easier it would be to grow a profitable clinic if you had more of those people on schedule.

How much easier would it be to raise your rates? How much better would your life be because you love to work with these people? Because they love to work with you? Because they pay you up front? Because it means that you can get home by 5pm each night as there's no insurance paperwork to spend hours doing at the end of the day?

This "ideal" person will have a certain type of injury they present with, they may be male or female, of a certain age, or they may even want to achieve a certain outcome such as playing golf or going back to cycling. Whatever it is, there will be a commonality that represents the "dream patient", a commonality that you want to see more of in your clinic.

Once you have that, the next thing to think about is that person's specific health challenges as well as the internal conflict that he or she has had to live with prior to coming to see you. Once you're clear on that, you need to talk exclusively about those two things in your marketing.

PAUL'S PERFECT PATIENT – SHE'S CALLED MARY!

At my clinic my perfect patient is a lady in her mid-50's. She values her independence and mobility, and she is frustrated at always being told by her local doctor to just "accept" her aches and pains as an "age thing". Often she is also fed up at being told to take some pills and come back in six weeks if it is no better (which it rarely ever is).

Those words are literally what she hears every time she goes to see her local doctor with something like back or knee pain, and because I am listening to her story, and paying attention to her, I am able to re-work the same words into my message to make an impact with her.

I call this lady "Mary" (she is based upon a real life patient). There is significance in knowing who she is and what her name is. It allows us to be able to make all of our business decisions with her in mind – marketing included.

Every single employee at my clinic will recall/mention her when they think about what they need to do to continue improving every aspect of our service. Knowing who this person is, and keeping a picture in my mind's eye, I can make better operational decisions all based upon how Mary would respond to what is happening or what we are about to do. The customer service is designed perfectly for Mary. The clinic's wall coloring, the waiting room material, the music on the internal speaker system, the candles, the coffee – these are all considered from the point of view of how Mary would feel about them. Would what we are about to do enhance or detract from our relationship with her? My hiring (and firing!) decisions get very easy, too. When I am looking at the candidate sat in front of me, I am able to close my eyes and ask myself the question: "will Mary love spending time with this person?" And then I'm guided by the answer.

WHY DID I CHOOSE MARY?

I chose a lady in her 50's for various reasons. To name just a couple, I chose her because females value their health more than men (broadly speaking, of course), they are used to spending money on themselves (to look and feel good), and a lady in her 50's now values her health a lot more than she did 10-15 years ago. All of this means that she is ultimately more open to paying to maintain it (I covered this in chapter 5 where I explained why the fortune is in the follow up). Plus, she is an "influencer". If I build up a great relationship with Mary then she is bringing her kids to see me, telling her husband he needs to come to the clinic, and I'll likely get her elderly parents too.

This is turning one patient into many, and this type of "home run" (where, thanks to Mary we get four patients coming to us very quickly) happens regularly. It gives me maximum return on my time and marketing money spent. I am getting significant leverage, and for all of those reasons it makes sense to focus on her more than anyone else.

BIRDS OF A FEATHER FLOCK TOGETHER!

Another great benefit of getting clear on your ideal patient is the fact that "birds of a feather flock together". I am sure you have heard the saying, and in this context what it means is that when you pick an ideal patient, you get to leverage the fact that they all hangout with other ideal patients who are just like them - people with the same values in terms of their health, and who are open to parting with the money it costs to maintain that health. We are not just looking for more volume of patients – that is easy – what we really want are people who value their health enough to pay for it, and at higher prices, enabling the running of a business. It justifies all the hassle and sacrifice that comes with running it.

I recall the first time I told my staff that we were narrowing down our audience to this ideal patient – singular – and to say that they were a little shocked is an understatement. I vividly remember thinking that they were looking at me as though I had "gone mad" and some were even worried that I was going to be downsizing the clinic and making people redundant. But, when I started to explain the principles behind the decision and the thought process that had gone into it, it all made sense to them.

Fast forward a few months after that meeting, my clinic was flooded with ladies in their 50's who were regularly telling us that their friends had told them about us.

Seriously, I remember sitting in the office out the back of one the clinics and looking at the waiting room, and every 30 minutes or so another "Mary" would walk through the door and sit on the couch. Your ideal patient is found in circles or communities with people who all value similar things. That is what a community or circle of friends is all about, it is why they exist. If you are doing a great job with your customer experience and the patient can really feel that the service you provide is "perfect for them", that it is what they want then they will tell similar people about you.

What they will say is that you are "perfect for people like us". The upshot is that when these people start calling your clinic there's no resistance to prices, and they agree to your plans of care because they are already pre-sold and bought in.

Think about how most clinics operate – it is the complete opposite. It is a case of "let's just set up shop and open the doors to anyone who will buy from us". That way of thinking might get you started, but it also gets you into a mess if it continues.

* I have added a video to the "resources kit" that accompanies this book; it shows you an interview that I did with the actual "Mary". It is footage of when she gave a testimonial for my clinic a few years back. Go to www.paulgough.com/resource to get this pack.

WHY I DIDN'T CHOOSE TO OPEN A SPORTS INJURIES CLINIC

Now I am not saying that you need to copy my ideal patient – what I am saying is copy how I came to the conclusion. Understand that I made a strategic decision. I looked around at what was happening in my area and realized that this particular person (Mary) was currently being underserved by the NHS (the free system), she was being overlooked by other clinics around me who were all marketing to the sports injuries crowd.

What I want to remind you of here is my background in professional soccer. I spent five years working with pro-soccer players, so I know how to rehabilitate ACL's, hamstrings, and ankle sprains etc., as well as anyone. My credibility in the pro-soccer game would have given me a distinct advantage over other clinics in the area, and most people assumed that when I left the pro-sport game I would open up a sports injuries clinic and focus on the athletes and gym goers – but I didn't.

I made a purposeful decision to focus on a group of people that, over and above all, had the fundamental attributes that you need from your patients if you want to grow a profitable business, the ability (financially), willingness (they want to do it!), and need (their problem is bad enough) to actually pay to have their health problem solved. The keys words (to have the patient actually pay) are **"ability"**, **"want"**, and **"need"**.

It is all well and good having the phone ring with inquires, but it is so much better when those inquires have the means to pay and are actually very happy to pay. But don't get me wrong, we still get the sports injuries. Soccer players, cyclists, and golfers all still find and choose my clinic. The point that I am trying to make is that in my town I accepted that there are not enough people with sports injuries who want to pay for my services, not if I wanted to grow and scale a business. If I existed solely in this market there would barely be enough business to cover my salary as a solo-practitioner – let alone all of the staff that I employ. In your area the sport injury market might be perfect for you. You need to determine what the right market will be for you to build and grow a profitable business.

With all of that said, go write down who the person is that you have identified, and then spend your whole career building a business just for them! By doing this, I guarantee that you've already gotten ahead of your competition and saved yourself years of heartache and struggle that comes with trying to get the wrong person to pay your fees.

STEP #2: GET THE RIGHT MESSAGE TO MARKET MATCH

The only way to make direct marketing work is to talk about their specific problems. At its heart your business is there to solve problems for people, and it is important that you understand how the person you are trying to market to sees her own problem. It is almost always very different from how we see it.

I have been quoted saying many times over, "it is not how we see it, only how they see it that matters". There's a particular "conversation" or internal dialogue that every one of your prospective patients is having, and you need to know what this sounds like so that you can market to them in a congruent way.

In marketing, (without getting too technical), it is simply called "entering the conversation in the persons head", and if you can do it (as in, step into it), you get significantly higher response rates from your ads, not to mention more compliance from your leads.

For example, that conversation a 55 year old might be having with herself (internal dialogue) could be about the fear that she is beginning to feel old. That fear could be brought on by the fact that a friend she hasn't seen in a while commented on how she might be moving a "little slower", or "not as well" as the last time they met. These are real conversations that happen every day, and despite what medical school might have taught you, these are the real drivers behind peoples' decisions to buy our services. This narrative is likely to be running through her head all day, every day. If you can come along with your marketing and speak to either of these things – slowing down or loosing energy as a result of back pain – then she is going to see that message and rightly assume that you know what she is living with, and very importantly, what she is going through. It is only when this happens that you get compliance and willingness to pay your fees.

Without doing step one (picking the perfect patient) we can never expect to do step two properly. Without knowing who your version of Mary is, you would be writing ads without any clear direction of what to say or who to say it to. That is the equivalent of being blindfolded and throwing darts at a board. The chances of hitting the board are very slim.

WHY AN 80 YEAR OLD FROM PHOENIX WAS HAPPY TO DRIVE 20 MILES AND PAY IN CASH

Remember when I told you earlier that people are motivated in different ways and that their motivation is mainly to solve some internal conflict (Chapter 5)? Well, here's a real life example of how truly understanding a person's real struggles and challenges makes acquiring new patients much easier:

A few years back I was writing a set of ads for a clinic in Phoenix. Because there are a lot of "seniors" and snowbirds living there (all wanting to be active and enjoy the warm weather), I chose to write the ad all about "maintaining independence" and "living a more active lifestyle free from pills".

A more active life and a better shot at maintaining independence was the **promise** that I was making in the ads. That was the marketing message. "If you want this (independence, mobility etc.), then I know how to get it for you, so call my clinic today."

As expected the phone rang off the hook from people wanting the "free tips report" we offered (showing them how to achieve it), one of the people who responded was a guy in his 80's…

What happened next is a very powerful demonstration of what I am saying here: when he called, the guy told the secretary that the reason he wanted the back pain report we were offering was because he was the "care provider" for his elderly wife. She was in a wheelchair and his health and ability to care for her was all that was stopping her from going into an assisted living home. This guy lived about 20 miles away from the clinic – a fair distance in Phoenix traffic - but even so, he was prepared to take the next step in the process and come in to the clinic to have a consultation with one of the physical therapists.

Not only was he willing to drive that distance, he was also willing to pay cash. The clinic did not take his insurance and they told him so on the phone – and yet he still wanted to come knowing full well he would be paying out of his own pocket **in cash.**

Think about this for a moment, he was willing to pay cash and drive 20 miles (passing by 5-10 clinics who would take his insurance), all because he saw an ad that spoke directly to his biggest fear – losing his independence.

This guy was willing to drive 20 miles and pay $150 in cash for this physical therapy service. Why was that? Surely that doesn't add up? Surely this guy under these circumstances would just go to the nearest clinic and get it for free (paid by his insurance)? He didn't do that. Instead he chose to drive and pay in cash with his own money. He <u>believed</u> that he was going to get something that the others couldn't offer. He believed that we would help to maintain his independence, and as a result, that we would improve his ability to continue to be a caregiver for as long as either he or his wife lived.

THAT was what he really wanted – the promise of an outcome that was made in the original marketing ad he had seen in the newspaper. That is how powerful this stuff is and why I'll never accept any clinic owner telling me that they can't make marketing work or that patients don't want to pay.

The reality is that if they are saying 'no', then they just don't want to pay for what is being promised or offered. The only option is to change it, and that is huge for you to understand (go back to chapter 5 for more on "Change the Meaning, Change the Outcome").

THE MESSAGE CHANGED - SO DID THE OUTCOME

Now I wish I could tell you that this story ended well – but it didn't. The guy in his 80's arrived for the session knowing full well what the costs would be moving forward, but he chose not to go ahead with a plan of care after the first session. Can you guess why?

It was because the therapist performing the initial consultation **stopped talking about independence** and instead, promised to ease the guy's back pain. The man was not there for relief of his back pain. He had lived with low-back pain for 30 years or more, so he did not think for one second anything could be done about it.

What he wanted (and what he was happy to pay cash for) was the hope that the pain would not get any worse. He wanted to be able keep active. There's a <u>big, big difference</u>. This principle is so misunderstood, and it is definitely not taught in those now very expensive PT Schools.

The therapist had the right intent, but the wrong execution. This physical therapist offered something that the patient could have gotten for much cheaper and with more convenience elsewhere (back pain relief).

Sadly, this type of thing is happening in clinics all day long. The lack of "message to market match" (spoke about in chapter 1) is the primary reason why clinics are struggling to get patients and compliance. Whatever you are saying and promising in your marketing has to be congruent with the person's desired outcome, or it'll fail. That is why you must spend some time figuring out what it is the patients really want or you'll keep on getting a "bad" response to your ads. In this case, the ads worked, but the $80k per year therapist didn't.

STEP #3: OFFER HELPFUL INFORMATION (TO START SOLVING THEIR PROBLEM)

So now that we know who they are and what their problems are, the next thing we need to do is offer them something to start solving those specific problems we identified above.

In chapter 1, I told you that one of the fundamentals to marketing success is the "offer" – the thing you want them to do or get from you. Well this is your version of that. The best way to do it is by giving them something like a "free tips report" (PDF/guide/report) that makes it less risky for them get in touch, thereby increasing response. The report starts to solve their problems and as a result, will give them what I call a "little win", giving them some confidence in you that you can help something be done for them.

It is important to make the first offer a "no-risk" one so that the patient cannot make a mistake by choosing you - offer a free report indicating that you are able to show them your familiarity with what their struggle is; offer to bridge the gap between where they are now and where they want to get to.

They are indecisive when they first see your ad. Where they want to get to is a better quality of life. At this point you might think that the thing stopping them from getting there is their pain or discomfort. But, it isn't. What *is* stopping them is their **inability to decide**. They cannot confidently decide on the best path of action to get to their end goal. This is a crucial distinction for you to make. Think about it, if they could decide, if they could make a decision, they would already be at their desired destination.

So, this indecision is actually presented as an opportunity you have to start helping them. Do not ask them to make a big commitment. Instead, be genuinely different from other physical therapists around you. Help build some confidence in their decision, some clarity about what is happening to them, and help them understand their choices and struggles.

Instead of asking them to walk across a "thin, icy lake" (that could crack and break at any time), why not build a steel bridge across to the other side, one that they can confidently place their first foot on and feel how safe it is? That is essentially what we are trying to do here. Instead of asking people to take a risk, make them feel safe and comfortable with every step they make with you. After each safe step they will feel more inclined to take another step, and another (and so on and so on) until they make their way into your treatment room and become a paying patient.

CREATE THE "TIPS" REPORT/PDF

This information report is going to be the front and central piece of your clinics marketing campaign. It'll contain information such as tips on best exercises, posture advice, educational classes they should consider, or it could even talk about how your great physical therapy skills can help patients. At this point we are not selling them an appointment – we just want them to be aware that you are an option.

This information could also be given to them in the form of a video or a book, but what I mostly use at my clinic is a free "tips" report, what is known as a 'lead magnet'. Something that, as the name suggests, magnetically attracts the right leads to your clinic (a working example of this lead magnet is included in your resource guide www.paulgough.com/resource).

It could be a report with a promise of easing back pain without needing surgery or pills. And the title of that report might be: "7 Ways To Ease Back Pain Without Taking Pills or Risking Surgery". In this report you will tell them seven very simple things to do. It doesn't have to be a "research" document fit for a medical department – just think, if your friend was out of town on vacation, and he hurt his back but couldn't get in to see you for treatment, what would you tell them to do? Whatever that would be, that is what goes into your tips report. You only need to tell them "what" to do. You do not tell them "how" to do… Why? Because if they want to know "how to do it", then they need to talk to you or hire you, which then becomes the logical next step. This is part of the conversion process from 'interested prospect', to that first consultation, and then to seriously considering hiring you.

WHY POSTING EXERCISE VIDEOS ON SOCIAL MEDIA IS A COMPLETE WASTE OF TIME!

Teaching the "why" (in your marketing), giving them the "what" (the free tips report), and selling them the "how" (your physical therapy services), is something very important for you understand. This is exactly how people buy. It is a logical sequence that starts with them understanding the "why" (the pain is happening to them), then learning the "what" (what can be done about it and by who), and finally understanding the "how".

A problem that I see in the profession is therapists skipping straight to the "how" phase by showing off their exercise videos on Facebook. The exercises are great, but the problem is they pre-suppose that anyone seeing them knows WHY they need to do them, and until you address that, they won't.

For example, have you ever told a five year old to put his coat on? Whenever I tell my son, Harry, to do something he immediately responds with "but why Daddy?" And no matter what I tell him he will repeatedly ask me "why" until he gets an answer he can understand or wants to hear.

The point I am making is that no one does anything until they understand the why. Your marketing talks to them about "why" they need to contact you. The message in the ad is all about their struggles and challenges and why they need to act now. That gets them motivated enough call to find out "what" they need to do, and this is where the video, DVD, book, or report comes in.

It doesn't need to be anymore than 5 minutes in length. In fact, any longer and it will get in the way of them taking the next step. If it's too long it will not get read. It will be left for another day or until they get time for it (which is never!). If they don't read it or watch it, then they don't get the chance to get that "little win". And we need them to experience that: it will mean they can start building some trust in you so that you can show them how you can help. Without this, they won't trust in themselves or that they can actually be helped.

MAKE AN EXCHANGE - YOUR EXPERT ADVICE FOR THEIR CONTACT DETAILS

At this point, all you have to do is motivate them just enough to make that first contact with you. You have to make the report title compelling enough for them to want to call your clinic or go online to get it.

What happens next is an "exchange". You will be swapping your great advice (contained inside the tips report or in the video) for their contact details. Getting their contact details is the "holy grail" in my business, it is the primary goal of this type of "relationship" marketing. Why is it so important to you? Because now you can use those contact details to keep in touch. You can call them back to ask if they have any questions they need answering before they hire you. You can even send them more information that you want them to read to help them believe you are the right choice and choose you.

This is called "nurturing", and it factors in that most people who see your ads are seeing you for the first time and they are considering you as an option for the very first time and his is important because hardly anyone buys things from anyone the first time they see or hear of a company or product (discussed in Chapter 1), especially not if the product is over $100 (as discussed in Chapter 5). And just because it is healthcare we are not exempt from that happening.

CONVERSION AND COMPLIANCE MADE EASIER

What this exchange also allows you to do is find out why people requested the free information. It allows you to find out "why didn't they want to hire you?" There is a reason that they chose the free and easy report, and that reason is the obstacle that stands in the way of them coming to see you. This exchange is your chance to find out what it is so that you address it and move onto the part where they get to become a patient!

When you stop and think about that question for a moment (...why did you choose a free report over getting specialist help from a physical therapist?) it tells you everything that you need to know about why the traditional sales model style advertising of qualifications and credentials does not work. People have obstacles and concerns, so until they are addressed directly those people will not come and see you no matter how qualified or experienced you are.

The point I am making here is that the exchange is vital. And it's not just about giving them information to start the journey with you – it's about creating a situation in which you are able to talk to people about what they want and what current concerns are getting in the way of hiring you. Just because they call and request information does not mean you have a patient. It means you have the initial commitment and attention of someone who lives close to you and who has a problem that you can solve – a qualified lead!

Now, just before we move on to create the system, let's recap the three steps we just covered:

1. **Pick your perfect patient (target market)**

2. **Work out their real problems so you can create the perfect marketing message and offer**

3. **Make an exchange – your free tips report for their contact details**

The next thing we are going to do is take these steps and put them into a marketing system – a lead generation and conversion system - that allows you to grow and scale predictably and profitably. Let's move on to chapter 7...

7

WHERE TO FIND AN ENDLESS SUPPLY OF YOUR PERFECT PATIENTS

So, now we know "who" the people are that you want to market to, as well as how to speak to the problems they are living with, the next thing that you need to do is to actually find them.

The final piece of the marketing triangle is the "media" or "platform" that you choose to run your ads on or in. There's a range of different marketing media available to you - social media, postcards, newspapers, Facebook, Google, and community events. The most important thing is to give some thought as to whether or not if, for example, you run a newspaper campaign, your perfect patient will see your ad. Will your 25-year-old CrossFit enthusiast, (your perfect patient), be looking there? Maybe. Maybe not. But I know it is more likely that a 60+ year old will be.

You can never be 100% certain, but when you spend at least some time asking yourself the question as to whether or not your prospects are using those platforms or looking there, you significantly increase your odds of marketing success.

INTRODUCING THE "ATTRACTION SYSTEM"

As I developed the "marketing machine" that fuels the growth of the Paul Gough Physio Rooms, I essentially broke it into three different systems

1. **Attraction System**

2. **Nurture System**

3. **Cash Value Maximization System**

Here's how they all fit together:

FIG.5

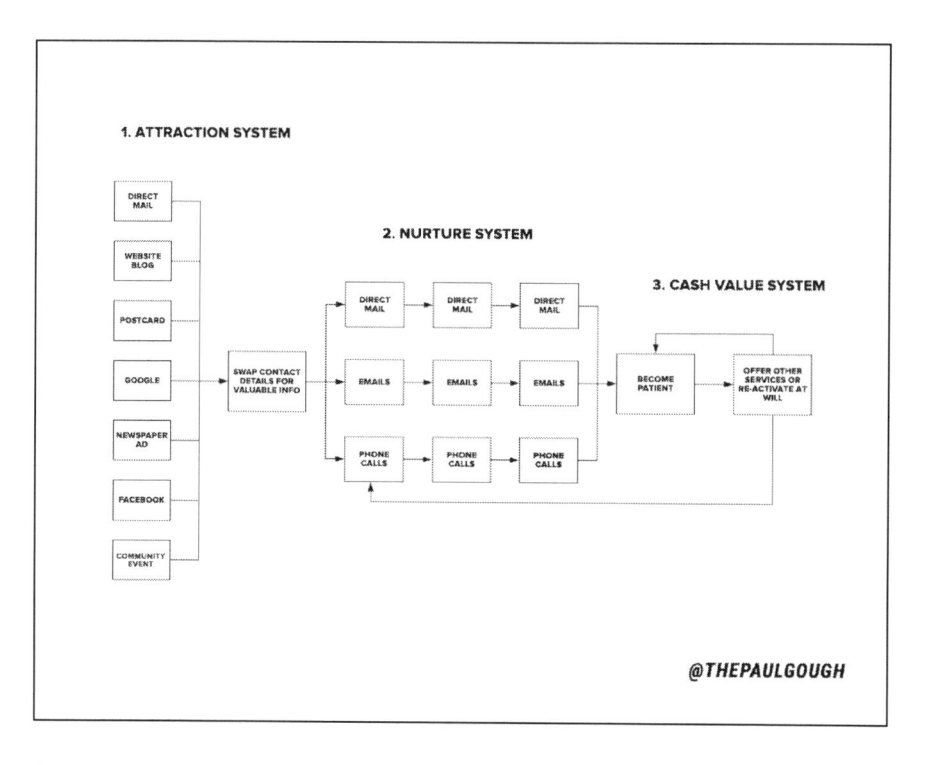

[Figure 5: Diagram showing the three interconnected systems – Attraction System (Direct Mail, Website Blog, Postcard, Google, Newspaper Ad, Facebook, Community Event) feeding into Swap Contact Details for Valuable Info, then into Nurture System (Direct Mail, Emails, Phone Calls in sequence), leading to Cash Value System (Become Patient, Offer Other Services or Re-Activate at Will). @THEPAULGOUGH]

As you can see, at the front of the Paul Gough Physio Rooms Marketing Machine is System 1 – The Attraction System.

All of them are inter-connected, but this is the one that starts everything off. It is the one that makes the phone ring in the first place, and it leverages all of the work you've done so far to pick your perfect patient, work out their real challenges and struggles, and what you've done to help them by creating the information needed to start solving their problems for them.

This system is all about getting seen by the right person. It leverages the different marketing media that we can use to put our message out there in front of the right person. **The Attraction System** is simply a means of targeting and attracting your perfect patient, and we do this through identification of her pain points, values, lifestyle, and health goals – and of course, her internal struggles and conflicts.

In the case of the 80 year old that I spoke about in the previous chapter, the internal conflict that he had was his worry over losing the ability to be the caregiver for his wife. He was more concerned with that than finding an end to his back pain. This Attraction System is your way of finding and then beginning a relationship with your perfect patients, showing them that you can solve their problems better than any other option they have. It is about positioning yourself as a specialized provider of solutions, helping patients understand that you know how to help them achieve their outcomes. It is not about "selling physical therapy", or even yourself and your experience, it is only about the outcomes that the perfect patient wants. If you take nothing else from this book, it should be that your marketing simply has to be about showing how you can solve specific outcomes that the patients want and are willing to pay for.

It is never about running an ad that says "call me today" or "book an appointment now". It's about running an ad that communicates your understanding of what they are going through and your willingness to help them figure out what the next best steps they need to make are – however long that takes.

To make this system work you need everything that we covered in the last chapter:

1. **The target market identified (perfect patient)**

2. The message that will resonate (what problem have they really got – usually internal)

3. The free report – give them a "little win" and start to solve their problems

Once you have those things you can then push on with selecting the media and running your new style ads.

Next let's look at five different examples of marketing media that you might use to run your new "Paul Style" ads as part of your Attraction System. I'll also break down how I've been able to make each of them work at my own clinic.

5 PROVEN NEW PATIENT ATTRACTION STRATEGIES

PATIENT ATTRACTION STRATEGY #1: NEWSPAPERS

Local newspaper advertising has become the backbone of my clinic's new patient attraction. It is a solid, consistent performer for the Paul Gough Physio Rooms that we quite simply never stop doing.

I know that many people close themselves off from this type of marketing because they don't read the newspapers, or they think that most people "do not read the newspapers" anymore. That simply isn't true. Sure, there might be less people reading them now than years gone by, but that's ok, we don't need everyone who was reading it, we just need a tiny percentage of the people who still are.

What is more, the fact that fewer people are now reading the newspapers means that it's cheaper than ever to get in there. Years ago, when all of the real estate, automotive companies and big law firms were advertising in the newspapers week after week, space was at a premium. It was almost impossible for a small company like you and I to advertise in there. But, these days all those companies are spending more of their ad budget elsewhere, whihcw means there's now more space. If there is less demand than supply, then it means prices are now more appealing to the likes of you and me.

I typically run 10" x 5", black and white, editorial style ads with compelling headlines. I have been able to pull in anything from 10-20 phone calls from one ad (*for an example of what one of my ads looks like, go to **www.paulgough.com/resource**, or join me for the online training and I'll walk you through how I create the ad: **www.acceleratorwebinar.com/book**). The great thing about newspaper ads is that the people who call are often easy to talk to and are generally very trusting and are open to hearing about the ways we can help them. The newspaper readers feel more confident and trusting because they've seen me in the newspapers week after week – they see me as a "local celebrity". Why wouldn't they? They continually see me in there.

BECOME A LOCAL CELEBRITY

I've had my picture in the paper so many times now that wherever I go people recognize me. They often stop me to tell me that an article I wrote resonated with them or to ask me a question about their health issues.

This is happening because the type of ads that I am running are a combination of what I call "tips" style, where I give simple and actionable health advice with a small call to action at the end asking readers to get in touch if they want more help from me, and true direct response ads (where I talk more about their problems, asking them to get in touch to claim a free report or book).

The cocktail of the two types of ads used regularly is not only bringing in more calls, but also has the added bonus of positing me as the "go-to" health expert in town, making conversion and compliance easier.

TRUST IS FOUND IN NEWSPAPER ADS

If you are sitting on the fence about advertising in newspapers, it might help you to understand that newspapers are still part of the original big "3" in advertising (TV and radio being the other 2).

What I mean by the "original big 3" is that these three media are still the ones that give you the highest level of authority and status if you are on, or in, any of them. The barrier to being seen or heard is high – your patients have been raised thinking that if you got on TV or radio then you were "famous", and if you were in the newspapers you did something very good or important (or really bad!).

I still remember the first time I appeared in the local newspapers – I was 18 and I had been selected to play cricket (the English version of Baseball) for my local county team. My dad rang me to tell me that I was in the paper and that people had called the house to congratulate me. The next day when I went to college, all of my friends had seen it and commented on it. I felt like a celebrity for the day, and it gave me a lot of attention.

That attention is something that can't be achieved from doing a "Facebook Live", or even putting something up on social media. I am not saying that you shouldn't do either of those two things, what I am saying is that there is a completely different level of trust when it comes to newspapers.

When people are considering buying from you, in the absence of trust and any other reason to do, they will always buy from the one that they have heard of. That is why famous people often charge a lot more than less famous people for the same thing or service.

Take Gordon Ramsey for example. He will demand at least two or three times more for the same fish that came out of the same ocean as his competition's fish. His cookbooks will sell for more than double his competition, and the demand for people wanting to get into his restaurants is a lot more than the one next door. Realistically, is the fish he serves any better than the one who's charging less? It might be. But most people will never find out. They just know that Gordon Ramsey is famous and therefore he must be better than the rest.

REVERSE ENGINEER REFERRALS

I've been teaching my clients to run newspaper ads for some time now and the impact that it has had on their businesses is staggering.

One of my clients, Dean Volk (mentioned in an earlier chapter). is located in Harrisburg, just outside of Charlotte; he also runs a cash based clinic in Charleston, South Carolina. He's gotten to the point where he's been seen in the local newspapers so often that patients are actually walking in to see their family doctor, pulling out the ad that they'd ripped from the newspaper on the weekend, and saying to the doctor, "I want a referral to this guy. This is the guy I want see. He seems to be the expert."

And why wouldn't they want to see him? He speaks all about their problems every week. He offers solutions to their problems every week. He offers them something of value (lead magnet/tips report) every week.

What Dean has done is **create demand** for his services, so even though he is a traditional insurance-based business in North Carolina, he is not having to go and knock on the doctors door and buy their lunch. He is getting the patients demanding that they are referred to him no matter where to, or to whom, the doctor tries to send them to. Even if the doctor tries to refer them to the bigger hospital systems or the physician owned clinics, they're still going to Dean because he's positioned himself as the expert - the "go-to" guy for back pain – in the whole of Harrisburg. That's the power of this type of marketing.

MORE PEOPLE TALKING ABOUT YOU = MORE REFERRALS

Newspaper advertising is also great for something called "pass along value." And what that means is that newspaper advertising makes it easy for people to tell others about you.

Here's a true story to explain what I mean: I have a client in Rochester Hills (MI), Oliver Patalinghug (of Restore PT), who I once wrote a series of low-back pain ads for, we were pulling in a great response right off the bat from being in the community newspaper every Wednesday. We were getting a steady 10-12 calls from people wanting his free tips report everytime we ran a 10" x 5" ad (costing approx. $300). He was converting 3-4 of them to paying patients very quickly. This was a good ROI. Then, he experienced the "pass along value", he started seeing patients come in because someone else told them about the newspaper ad and they wanted to see the guy who was "in the paper."

"MY MOM TOLD ME TO COME AND SEE YOU"

I remember one specific example of this is when he was treating a guy in his mid-30's. This guy had been to see his local doctor and asked for a referral to Oliver. Yet when he called Oliver's clinic he told the receptionist that he was referred by his doctor. Of course, technically, he was. But what or who was responsible for the referral request? Well, about two weeks into the treatment plan the guy said something to Oliver that made him realize just how powerful his ads were and how much impact they were really having.

The patient told Oliver that his mother enjoys reading his article every week, and that he only booked the appointment because his mother (in her late 60's) reads the articles. She told him that he should see "this guy". Not a physical therapist, but "this guy"! **Big difference.**

It said "doctor referral" on the new patient register, but the reality was that the newspaper had caused a conversation between him and his mother, and that conversation led him to asking the doctor to send him to Oliver. The newspaper ad was the **first touch** that kicked the referral process off. Had Oliver not been in the newspaper, had he not been seen by the patient's mother, chances are that the guy would still be suffering now. Alternatively, he would have been sent somewhere other than Oliver's clinic.

NEWSPAPER ADS KEPT IN GOLF BAGS!

This is not a one off. I've heard this type of story many times at my own clinic as well as at others that I work with. Another client of mine had a similar experience, Andrew Vertson of Intecore PT in Orange County, California. I once wrote him a series of back pain ads aimed at targeting golfers in the area. And one day, a few months after the already successful campaign had finished, a guy turned up in his clinic holding onto a "cut-out" of the same ad that had been in the paper months before. The patient said that his friend from the golf club noticed the ad, had kept it for him, and gave it to him knowing he was suffering with back pain and struggling to play golf. The patient had kept the cut out of the ad in his golf bag for two months, only to call it in when his back pain got so bad that he couldn't make it past the 4th hole.

Pass along value is huge. It means that newspapers give you many more things than most other platforms can. You get leads in the short term, you get credibility and authority which makes conversion and compliance easier, and you also get long-term success from the people who see you, keep your ad, and use it when they are ready to call.

If I remember correctly, this patient even asked Andrew to "sign" his autograph his free report for him. In the mind of the patient, Andrew was a **local celebrity.** How hard do you think Andrew had to work at getting this guy to comply or pay his fees? Not very, is the answer.

PATIENT ATTRACTION STRATEGY #2: FACEBOOK

Let's move from "offline" to "online". Facebook advertising is something that I've been doing at my practice since the day it became an option, back in 2013.

I've since spent in excess of $100,000 on Facebook – and that's because it works! It is a platform that is difficult to hide from and I don't know many, if any, niches or perfect patients that you wouldn't be able to find from advertising on Facebook. It's great for getting leads and raising general awareness of who you are and what you can to do help people.

I primarily use Facebook ads to get leads and build my celebrity status and authority. It is not about selling things or asking people to commit to appointments. It is not about asking for likes or even worrying over things getting shared. It is all about positioning yourself and getting leads that will go through your Nurture System (discussed in the next chapter).

To be clear, what we are talking about here is Facebook's paid for ad platform. It is NOT about posting status updates and images. It is about paying for your ads to be seen by the people in your target market. And that is what makes Facebook so special and unique. Facebook's ad platform allows for great targeting so it is very easy to find your perfect patient – you could easily find guys in their 30's who like to do CrossFit, or ladies in their 50's who want to be active and enjoy yoga.

If you are in the postnatal back pain or pelvic floor niche, you could very easily find ladies who have just given birth or are about to. You could even talk to middle-aged children who are worried about their elderly parents falling. For all those reasons, Facebook cannot be ignored. I have mainly targeted ladies in their 50's and above. This allows me to write the message in the ad specifically for that person who's living with a certain type of problem (…an example of one of my best Facebook ads is in your resource kit **www.paulgough/resource**).

Because I know the ad will only be seen by ladies in their 50's, I make the ad specific to them – and only them – and this makes the chance of getting a response higher. I might say something like: "Ladies, are you fed up of trying to live an active life in your 50's – always being held back from enjoying it by low-back pain that won't seem to shift?"

This is an incredibly powerful message to a lady in her 50's, it strikes a chord with the person seeing it, and that makes them instantly think that I understand them (which I do!). It would not resonate with a guy in his 20's, but that is ok, he is not going to see it. With this type of message, I am entering the conversation inside the person's head (discussed in chapter 6), and this causes her to "agree" with me, to say "yes, I have had enough!" The moment they privately acknowledge that, they are more likely to take the next step to becoming a lead, and then converted to a patient.

MAKING FACEBOOK WORK

Here's a few tips for getting Facebook right: first, recognize that there is a big difference between posting on your personal or business pages, and advertising on the Facebook Ads platform. Expanding your social network on Facebook is important, but if you gave me the option of paying for ads to be served into the newsfeeds of my perfect patient, or constantly posting to my personal account, I'd pay, all day, every day. When all is said and done, as business owners, we are in the business of **multiplying capital by leveraging assets** - and your marketing message is an asset.

If you truly understand who it is you want to work with, and you're able to speak to them in a way that will resonate with them like no one else, then you should not be worried about spending money on Facebook. Take advantage of its incredible targeting capabilities which narrow down your audience so that fewer people see your ads more often. Do not look to sell anything directly from Facebook - it is 100% about raising awareness of the fact that you exist and that you know how to solve the patient's problem.

Some of my best paying patients started out watching a video that I posted on the Facebook Ads platform. They later went onto request a free report, then they went into my **Nurture System**, and finally they became a high paying patient. When it comes to automating leads, Facebook is one of the very best ways of doing it.

PATIENT ATTRACTION STRATEGY #3: DIRECT MAIL AND POSTCARD MARKETING

Let's go back "offline" and talk about sending direct mail or postcards to your perfect patient. I have had great success with direct mail campaigns; I like them because they are quick and easy to get started, and in most instances they can be very cost effective.

We'll start with postcard marketing. The first thing to remember is that we don't want to be mailing anyone and everyone in your town. You only want to be mailing your perfect patient. You will be more successful by mailing 100 of your perfect patients than 1,000 people at random. Go deep, not wide. This requires you to have a list of people who represent your ideal patient: there are many services that allow you to go online and search for your perfect patient by their demographic and geographic location.

For example, I could talk to a "list broker" and rent or buy a list of 500 people living within five miles of my clinic. I could get even more specific by ensuring that the list of names and addresses I got within that five mile radius only contained females in their 50's, and, that each household has more than four people in the house. That would suggest that the lady has two children and that she is family orientated. That is the person who I know is likely to spend more money with me. I could get even more specific and ensure that the person had an average household income of $100,000 or more. I could even rent or buy a list of people who fit all of those criteria and additionally, have recently bought some kind of health product in the past 12 months.

Again, as you are reading this you are seeing that the success of any direct marketing lies in knowing "who" your perfect patient is. Even with postcards and direct mail, you must know who that person is, if you don't, **marketing to them is not going to work.**

HOW TO MAKE POSTCARD MARKETING WORK

So, to make this work I must first get a list (from a local list broker, or online) which contains all of the names and addresses of the people I want to target. Start with no more than 300-500 names. I once heard a story of a physical therapist sending 12,000 pieces out – the campaign failed spectacularly. That is like burning $12,000 right in front of your eyes.

That's not fun. It would have been obvious after mailing 500 that the campaign wasn't going to work and he could have altered the message before the next 500 went out.

The smart way to do it is to start with an initial 300-500 names. Mail these people a 6" x 11" (oversized) postcard that talks to them about their problems and how you are familiar with them. Then, "offer" them something that they can get from you in the way of starting to solve that problem. What might that "offer" be? Of course, it is going to be your lead magnet (free tips report).

If you are targeting people with back pain and you have a list of 500 people aged 50 and above, then there is a very good chance that 50 or so will currently have back pain or suffer from it regularly. And in the same way as newspapers work, the person who you send the postcard to will most likely know someone else who suffers from low back pain she will kindly show or give the postcard to them.

DIRECT MAIL - JUST AS EFFECTIVE

Really, the only difference between postcards and direct mail is the format. The content hardly changes. Sure, there might be slightly fewer words on a postcard, but what you are saying and offering is not all that different. Fewer words, but the same message.

My secret is to always start a marketing campaign using the longest piece I need to write - I take out the main points of the letter and copy it across to create a postcard. And if you want to know how I get the content for my letter, it comes from the newspaper ad content that I write. I am not re-inventing the wheel here. I am not writing for the sake of writing. I am just taking what I know works best and putting the same message onto a different marketing media. If people respond to the newspaper ad, it tells me that the message works: all I have to do now is roll it out across the different media.

The point is that people respond differently to different marketing media. Someone might like to read it in a long-form letter. The person next door might not have the time to read that length, and instead prefers to read it in a shorter form like a postcard. This is vital for you to understand because really, all you have to do is commit to getting one of these media right. Once you know the person, you've got the message in the ad right, and the offer is pulling in phone calls, you can very easily move it to another platform. It is called the **"Wheel of Engagement"**, whereby you take the same piece of engaging content and get it seen everywhere your perfect patient is looking.

To sum it up - the most important thing to get right when it comes to making postcard and direct mail work is…drum roll please… the target market - the "list" you will buy or rent, and use. If you do not have the right people on that list, those who resonate with your headline, or your marketing message is weak and the offer of the free report is not able to solve their problem, then they will not respond (no matter how nicely it is designed or how big your logo is).

Postcard marketing and direct mail can also be used to market to your past patients. As a general rule, I make a point of marketing to my past patients by mail at least once per month. Never let anyone tell you that the old school stuff is dead – I assure you I would not be spending my money on it if it didn't work.

PATIENT ATTRACTION STRATEGY #4: GOOGLE ADWORDS (PPC)

Google AdWords (also known as Pay Per Click or "PPC") was the very first marketing strategy that I studied and implemented. It was the platform that, quite literally, exploded the number of calls I was getting. And it happened almost overnight. Google AdWords puts you right, slap bang in front of people actively looking for the service that you can provide. It puts you no.1 on the most respected and used search engine in the world and yet despite all of its well know advantages and benefits, most physical therapists will never get to experience any of them!

Let me explain: Google AdWords is the express route to getting your website found. It is without a doubt the nut-to-crack if you want to get more call from hot prospects, quickly. At the time of writing, I have spent in excess of $200,000 on Google AdWords and it has produced a return of well over $1,000,000. That amount is figured solely by the amount of patients I have gotten from it and how much they've spent with me. I love giving Google as much of my money as possible.

Now, if you are unfamiliar with Google AdWords, you will likely have used it as a consumer. These Google ads are the first three or four options that you see at the top of the search you have just performed on Google. If you search for "Villas in Hawaii", you'll see that the first few choices are a slightly different color from the ones below. How it works is that companies pay or "bid" to be in the top 1, 2 or 3 positions (to avoid getting stuck lower down the page where no one looks).

However, most business owners choose to rely upon the free listings (because it is free), and the fact that it's free is precisely the problem. If it is free, everyone who's running a physical therapy clinic in your town is also in there, making it harder to get seen or noticed. When people call up and ask for your price they are literally going through all of the providers in the free listings on Google. By appearing in the free listings only, you have let yourself become a commodity.

GET TO NO.1 ON THE WORLDS BIGGEST ADVERTISING PLATFORM

Getting to no.1 on Google gives you a big advantage in that you are positioned as an authority. It is like you are being endorsed by one of the most successful companies in the world, and it adds a lot of weight to your authority and superiority in the eyes of the prospective patient.

Google Ads often work rapidly, because unlike on Facebook, in newspapers, or even in postcard marketing, the person is looking for you. It is attraction marketing at its very best, and is the best option there is if you want to get in front of people searching for help to problems you can solve - fast.

What I love about Google AdWords is that it is a lot like a tap that I can turn on and off when I want. Meaning, if we are at capacity in one clinic then I can turn my entire ad budget to a clinic that is slightly quieter. If we are busy across all clinics, I can ease off on the ads. If we are quiet in all clinics, I can turn the ads back on, and within an hour I am number No.1 on Google again. It is very powerful and an incredible tool to have in your marketing kit.

TIPS TO GET TO NUMBER 1 ON GOOGLE

To make this strategy work you have to follow the rules of everything that I have taught you so far. If you know who your perfect patient is and that they are likely to be living with, for example, 'back' or 'knee' pain, then you can set up your Google AdWords account to trigger an ad for your clinic when someone types in the words "ways to ease back pain", or "how to ease knee pain" (both of which would be very common).

You get the luxury of great targeting options as well. Google gives you geo-targeting, which basically means that the ad will only pop up when someone is within a certain radius of your clinic (which you can set), and the best bit is this - you only pay for the ad when they click on the ad. If they don't click – you don't pay.

Think about what that means – it is like negotiating a deal with the local newspaper that says you only have to pay if someone calls you. With that type of deal you would never stop running the ad because you would have nothing to lose. It is the same with Google Ads. If you have done your targeting right, you've created a compelling first ad, and your website is designed to talk to your perfect patient, then you will have no problem with getting a return from Google.

Not many people understand this, but Google is ultimately a "question engine" that people go to when they want answers. Your prospects are right at this moment asking Google a question to try and solve their health and fitness problems. And if used correctly, Google will assist you by putting you in front of those people who are actively looking. That, right there, is the no.1 problem in most businesses solved.

BUT MOST WEBSITES ARE NOT DESIGNED TO BE SUCCESSFUL ON GOOGLE

I've just told you how great Google AdWords is. Now, here's the bad news. Most websites are not set up to support being successful on Google. That is because, like most traditional marketing methods, they are designed to sell the credentials and experience of the clinic owner. It is designed to look nice, and in the hope that it looks attractive enough, the owner believes it'll convince the onlooker to book an appointment with him.

Here's a reality check about websites: there are significantly less people are looking for physical therapy than those that are looking for back pain or knee pain advice. Yet, almost every one of the physical therapy website companies out there insists on creating a website all about you and physical therapy? It is madness. Yet, it also explains why so many people are left so frustrated by their websites. They are designed to sell physical therapy when they should be designed to start a relationship, to provide helpful information to start solving someone's problem. If you want to make Google AdWords work, you must have a website that offers information, it must be an avenue which gives people the option to book an appointment with you. If you do not do that, your website will be a complete waste of time and money.

How can I be sure that most websites are a complete waste of money? Well, Google provides data on the searches being done in your area, specifically those that are relevant to your website. When I looked at the number of times someone was searching for "ways to ease back pain", I found that it was 100x more than anyone searching for "physical therapy in Hartlepool" (where one of my clinics is based).

To put that into context, that means for every single person searching for physical therapy in Hartlepool there are 100 more looking for help with their back pain. Your website must factor this in, otherwise you'll be losing out on a huge volume of patients who need you. (*I've put an example of one of my Google Ads in your resource PDF at **www.paulgough.com/resource**).

PATIENT ATTRACTION STRATEGY #5: COMMUNITY EVENTS, SCHOOL FAIRS, AND CHURCH FAIRS

Getting to local community events, school fairs, EXPOS, and being at the finish line of a 5k run ("tents at events"), are great ways to find and begin very strong relationships with high value patients. Doing this type of thing is no different from running an advert in the local newspaper or on Facebook – you are going to <u>position yourself as an expert who provides solutions to specific problems.</u>

In this case, your attraction magnet is the booth, table, or stall that you take. You are going to follow the exact same strategy and principles that I've taught you previously. Your ad, in this instance, would be the message that is displayed on your stall or the pull-up banner that you would position either side of the table.

DON'T MAKE IT ABOUT YOU

The big mistake is to think that you go to these events to make it all about you and your clinic. I've been to many open air markets and school or church fairs (as a visitor), and walked past many local physical therapists or chiropractors attempting to bring people to his stand, often by offering something like a "free massage" or a "free screen".

This is pretty standard in our profession. The therapist has great intentions and is hoping that tons of people will come over and start talking to him because of these. The problem with this strategy is that it scares most people off much more than it will ever attract them.

Sure, some people will come over to the stand if you position the booth to be all about you and your clinic, but only those who know what you do, and only those seriously considering going forward, will seek some help. Which is very few people.

It is much better to turn that stall or booth into an "information booth" where people can walk over to you and get information on solving a problem that they might have.

What you want to come away with when doing this type of event is a collection of qualified leads. Once you get leads you can let your **Nurture System** (discussed in the next chapter) take over and do the job of converting those leads into paying patients. If the booth is positioned as a place that people can walk over to, free from the worry of having to possibly make a big commitment with you, then you will increase the number of people who come over by at least 10x.

You will still be getting the people who might want a free massage or a free screen (offer it to them for coming over, just as a surprise bonus), but most importantly of all, you will get all of the people who didn't want either and who are actually put off by the prospect of being sold to whilst being there with their families and having a pleasant time.

If you position yourself as an expert, someone happy to provide valuable information, then you are following the rules of the Accelerator Method and you're using lead generation and education based marketing strategies to their full effect. Instead of the typical banner saying "Paul Gough Physio Rooms", the banner's message should say: "If you have knee or back pain – walk over here to get your free information booklet".

I am talking to them about their external pain point, and when they walk over to get the free information booklet (the lead magnet/PDF), then I am going to continue the conversation and ask questions that lead them to telling me more about their internal conflict and struggle. When they tell me this, I am then in a position to match up how my skills can help solve those specific problems.

Now because you now know who your perfect patient is, you can start asking yourself good questions about whether or not they would be at such a thing as a Sunday open air market or upcoming community event. You would approach this scenario in the exact same way as Facebook or a newspaper ad. There's no guesswork in this anymore; you can be more confident about making the investment or commitment to go and do it.

For example; if some of your best patients all send their children to a certain school in town, and that school is running a fair next month, then you know it is going to be a great way to get in front of other people who are likely to be very similar to your perfect patient. Remember, birds of a feather flock together - and birds of a feather often have similar values, lifestyle and health goals.

Getting to these types of events, and using your stall as an "attraction magnet" by positioning yourself as a trusted provider of advice and information is smart, and it is no different to doing it on the other media or platforms we've run through. Instead of asking people to commit to booking "free screens", or "free massages", you are saying, "hey, come over here if you need some information on back pain". You are saying, "let me help you first", and "let's get to know each other", and then, who knows, it may be that after 10-15 minutes of talking to them they then want to take a free screen, or better yet, book an appointment with you.

It's my experience that the more time I spend with prospective patients at these types of events, the better type of patient they become. There's a direct relationship between the time I spend listening to them during the conversation and the compliance that I get. The more I give them, the more they give me.

"PAUL IS EVERYWHERE" - OMNIPRESENCE

I have just given you five examples of how you can make the Accelerator Method work. You are taking 3 solid principles (pick your perfect patient, work out their internal problems, offer them information to build a bridge), and all you are doing is taking the same information and replicating it across any of the 10, 15 or 20 potential different media or platforms that you could be advertising to your perfect patient on.

To get going, just commit to starting with one of these platforms or media and then build on it as the results come in. For example, as the revenue starts to flow in, having advertised in the local newspapers, take some of it and spend it on Facebook. You now have two ads running, and when the revenue comes back in from the Facebook ad, spend it on a monthly postcard. As the money from that comes in, you can spend it on getting started with Google AdWords. And then, when that starts to come in, you use that money to get a regular spot at a local community event or school fair. This is how you will create something called "omnipresence", which is basically a situation where people are seeing you **everywhere**.

At the Paul Gough Physio Rooms, at any one time we could have seven or eight different marketing strategies in place; these might include email, remarketing, social media, letters being sent to past patients, as well as all of the things I've just described above. This means that no matter where my patients look – I am there. Heck, because of my book (The Healthy Habit) they are even seeing me on Amazon!

"I AM SICK OF SEEING PAUL'S FACE!"

Writing about omnipresence reminds me of a story. A patient who spent weeks deliberating over whether or not she should come to see me eventually got so sick of seeing my face that she quite literally, "gave up!"

This lady would walk past my clinic in Guisborough every day on her way to work, and secretly she knew that she needed to come and see me. But she was always "contemplating it" and would never quite get round to doing it (like so many). She privately admitted that she knew from that first day of seeing my clinic that she needed to see me – yet she continued to delay coming in, constantly finding some excuse not to do it, and always telling herself that tomorrow she would be ok.

It was while walking past my clinic that she noticed a picture of my book, The Healthy Habit, advertised in the window. As the story goes, she decided to go online and look at it later that day. She looked in two places - firstly she looked on Amazon, and secondly, she looked on the official website (the website I own which officially sells it). Because she did this (went to my website and Amazon), a couple of things happened; one of them was she that was tracked in my clinic's "remarketing" ad campaign (also known as cookies), a feature we use to market to people across the internet who have visited any of my sites. How it works is like this: when you visit my website I will continue to show you an ad for my clinic for up to six months, or until you fill out a form on my website that indicates you have made an inquiry with me.

This lady was now seeing these ads advertising my clinic, but because she had also looked at my book on Amazon - though hadn't purchased it yet – she was also seeing my face on an ad from Amazon every time she went online to shop with them. (Amazon has the same remarketing cookies set up as we do, and that explains why you will always see images of things you have looked at, but haven't bought yet).

EMAIL MARKETING KICKED IN AFTER SHE BOUGHT THE BOOK

Now eventually she did buy the book. And she bought it via the official website (of The Healthy Habit), which means she was now a customer of mine and was getting emails from me (because she gave me her email address).

So at this point she is now seeing me all over the Internet whenever she goes online or opens her emails, and I'm likely to be the last thing she sees before bed (as she reads a chapter of the book that she bought each night).

Next, she picks up the local newspaper in Guisborough and when she gets to page 17, guess who she sees a picture of? Of course it is "yours truly" talking about back pain struggles – her back pain struggles (that is four media she is now seeing me in)! Yet, she still resists calling and making an appointment.

Next she goes to Facebook and guess who she sees there? Of course, it is me in a video talking about low back pain and how to fix it. As I told you above, Facebook's targeting means that I am able to show my videos to ladies in their 50's and 60's who live within a 10 mile radius of my Guisborough clinic. This lady was right in that bracket (that is the fifth marketing media she has seen me on).

Next, because I had her address (because she bought the book directly from me) I was able to send her a letter offering her a chance to come to the clinic for an educational class to learn more about back pain and how we could help her.

At this point I was now in her inbox, in the newspapers she was reading, on Amazon when she shopped there, on every Internet page she was looking at, in her Facebook newsfeed, and now I was in her mailbox – that is six different marketing media (not to mention my clinic, which she walked past every day; it has a sign outside saying "come in if you are worried about back pain").

I was everywhere this lady looked, and collectively, all of these different marketing media, each showing her the same marketing message, promising to solve her problem, caused her to make the decision and book a physical therapy appointment with me in the end. Who knows which one was the "straw that broke the camel's back". There's never one single chop with the axe that causes the tree to fall. It is the same in marketing – it is the total of all of the activity resulting in the decision to finally say yes. The more times you swing the axe, the faster the tree will fall.

What is funny is that when she did eventually book the appointment she told my front desk person that she "gives up!"; in her own words, "she was sick of seeing my face everywhere she looked". Apparently, she felt that in the end seeing my appearance everywhere "was a sign". **It was a sign** – a sign from me that she needed to get the appointment booked!

I have lost count of the number of times I have heard a story like this at my clinic, and the moral of the story is that being in one place is better than being in no place. The moment you can get to the point of advertising in different places simultaneously is when your clinic is really going to get to the next level.

Never mind looking to save money on marketing, you should always be <u>looking to spend more</u>. "Paul Style" marketing is about spending as much money as you possibly can (and not spending less), but doing so in a way that means you are always making more money than you are spending on advertising.

Never forget that the purpose of a business is to turn **assets** into **revenue,** and **revenue** into **profit** – and that **profit** into **cash**. Your marketing is what drives the revenue you need if you are to have a chance at making a profit. Said differently, if you do not invest in your marketing, you will never create revenue and you'll never make a profit – and you can forget about having cash in the bank to spend or take home.

Be careful of how you perceive your marketing spending - it should not be as an "expense". Done right, it does not cost you any money at all, and the more you spend, the more you should make. Your accountant might disagree, but that is because he believes, often falsely, that the only way to grow a business is to cut costs. I remember when I first employed my own in-house financial controller to look over all the revenue that was flowing through my four businesses, and at the end of the first year he was employed, he looked on in amazement at the amount I had spent on marketing.

He suggested that next year I might want to cut down on that marketing expenditure, and if I did, we would make more money. I politely reminded him that the only reason he had a job with me was because of the money I spent on marketing – and the revenue it brought in. If I cut down on marketing I would also have to cut his position. Needless to say, he was happy to see my marketing expenditure from a different point of view.

So now that you've got your leads coming in from various sources, let's look at how you are going to convert them to paying patients who are happy to comply. Remember my story from earlier in the book about how the "fortune is in the follow up"? Well, in the next chapter we will be creating your follow up machine - that is the second of the three systems you need, and is what I call the **"Nurture System"**.

8

HOW TO GET PAID FASTER – TURN INQUIRIES INTO HIGH PAYING PATIENTS FAST

In the previous chapter you learned how to create an Attraction System to get more people to call you. The next thing you need is a system to convert those people into high paying patients.

I call this the **Nurture System.** The Nurture System is connected to the Attraction System and sits in the middle of your clinics marketing machine. Here's how it looks:

FIG.6

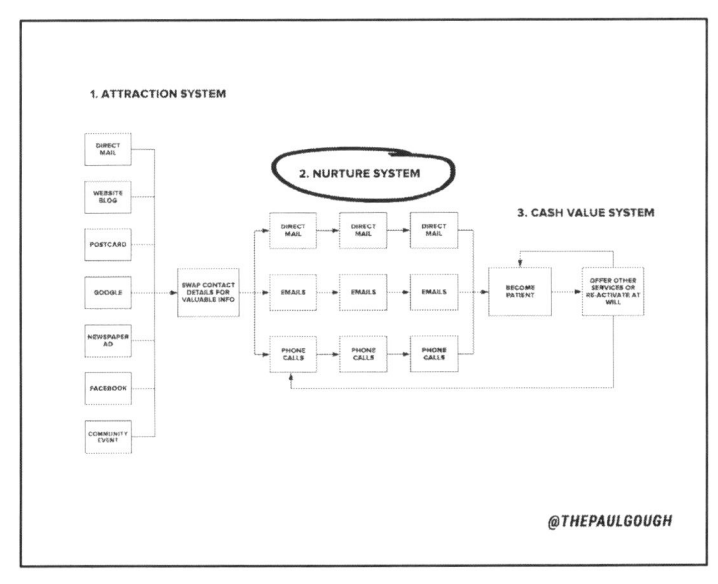

As you look at the flow diagram you can see that people start with you on the left having responded to one of your ads, a report is then exchanged, and finally they move through to the Nurture System where you start the process of converting them to becoming a patient.

The Nurture System is the critical link between people who make inquires in response to your ads - and you getting paid.

With your Attraction System in full swing you are going to get calls from people interested in getting a solution (to their problems). At this stage they are "leads". They've called you, but there's no real understanding of what you do yet. Until that is addressed, it is going to get in the way of conversion and compliance. The people who are calling you are interested and curious about what you can do for them; your Nurture System will take them all the way from 'interested' to committed and happy to pay for your services.

The Nurture System is made up of things like phone calls, emails, and direct mail; these start immediately after a prospect requests your free report. It is a mostly **automated system** that allows you to find out what people want from you so that you can educate them on how you can provide it. So that they are more likely to want to book an appointment with you.

To be clear: the potential patient requesting a report is step 1. Step 2 is following up with them until they are ready to book, and it is this that is the missing link for most businesses. If they had this type of Nurture or "Follow Up" System in place, they would likely double, or even triple their patient volume. It certainty changed everything for me.

THE BEST ROI ON MY TIME - EVER

As I write these words (from a coffee shop in Memphis, TN), there are literally thousands of people going through my clinic's Nurture System right now, each receiving communication from me that I created years ago. The point I am trying to make is that even though I am writing these words in Memphis – some 4,000 miles away – my potential patients are being nurtured by this system.

To this day, there's been no better ROI in terms of my time than I invested in creating this second system. And having it automated gives me tremendous leverage. This means I can do more, with less (i.e. I can write this book and build a second business while my clinic continues to grow).

If you have an automated system for converting your patients it means you spend more time actually running the business, leaving it safe in the knowledge that the most important aspect of the business is taken care of - the patient actually saying yes to paying for the treatment, and of course, you getting paid.

THE POWER OF HAVING A PIPELINE

When people start to call you (having seen your compelling attraction ad) you will create a "pipeline" for those leads. This pipeline is the breathing space that most clinic owners never have. Most clinic owners are waking up today, hoping and praying that the phone is going to ring from the folks in Group 1 ("ready to buy now"). Yet the **freedom**, the **wealth**, and the ability to **sleep at night** and to not have to sweat about making pay-roll at the end of the month, that only comes from having leads in a pipeline (Group 2, explained in Chapter 1).

If the phone stops ringing at my clinic, if people aren't asking for appointments (Group 1 – "ready to book now") – no problem. We have more time and can put more effort into developing the leads in our pipeline (Group 2). Instead of staring at the phone, hoping and praying it will ring, we are picking up the phone and making something happen. We are being proactive instead of passive.

It also turns my admin staff into revenue generators. Instead of my office staff tidying up or shuffling paper all trying to look busy, they are being productive, doing something to bring in revenue so that I can pay the bills and make a profit that justifies actually being in business in the first place.

Because people leave us their phone number, email, and sometimes their address when they request free reports, it means that my staff can be on the phone as soon as it goes quiet. By the end of a day that might have been a "bad one" as far as new patients go, we've converted leads from our pipeline and everyone is getting paid at the end of the month - without worry.

That is a very powerful position to be in. And is the complete opposite of most business owners who are relying on a fax coming in from a doctor or the phone to ring from a past patient.

THE MORNING MADNESS OF A TYPICAL CLINIC

Think about a typical day in a typical clinic likes ours; the phone, if it is going to ring at all, will usually ring early on in the morning. Typically, the callers will be patients who decided the previous day or night that they need to call and finally make an appointment. By midday, the early morning "mad-rush" for appointments is over and the rest of the day is for processing invoices or catching up on paper work, etc.

Not in my office. When the morning rush is over and people have stopped calling "in", my staff are calling "out". They are talking to leads. We are affecting the day actively. We are making a difference on bad days, always limiting the baron spells that so many clinic owners believe they have to accept as though it is somehow normal.

If there is anything that you take away from this book, it should be the importance of turning your business from one that is passive and waiting for the phone to ring (always relying on doctors or word of mouth), to one that is pro-active and able to make outbound calls, booking people in if and when it goes quiet.

If you are always waiting for the phone to ring and it doesn't, and you have no pipeline to go-to to make a bad day great, then your clinic will always be stuck in the "boom and bust" scenario that we spoke about earlier in the book. I do not like the thought that my clinic's profit, and my ability to pay my mortgage, are at the mercy of whether or not someone may or may not talk about me today. It is a very vulnerable place to be in as a business owner. It's much better to have leads in a pipeline, ones you can go to and talk to if, and when, your phones go quiet.

LEADS CONVERT AT DIFFERENT TIMES – AND THAT'S OK

The leads in your pipeline will all convert at different times. Some are ready to go within days and some might take 12 months, and this is why we have a Nurture System; when you have a lead that is ready to convert, you are the only clinic that she thinks of.

If the pipeline is constantly filled, you'll find that soon after the process starts it is absolutely reliable. On the same day a new lead is entered, you'll already have access to several that were added 3 weeks ago, all of who will convert to paying patients! It obviously takes time for the first batch of leads that you put into your pipeline to convert, but pretty soon after you start you will find that you have new patients converting at the same time as you are adding new leads.

It's been five plus years since I started this at my clinic and I still have people who might take 12 months to covert – and others that convert right away. What matters most is not when they convert, it is only that they do! **"You will be my patient, we just have not agreed on a date and time"** is the mindset I have adopted. I recommend you do the same too.

I've learned that the longer it takes for the patient to convert the more compliant they are, they are more bought in to what we can do for them. This is one of the reasons that I am, to my knowledge, one of the highest charging physical therapy clinics in the whole of the UK (possibly THE highest!).

WHAT TO PUT IN THE FOLLOW UP SYSTEM

The aim of this system is to provide the patient with educational information to help them make a better, more educated, and more informed decision about hiring you and choosing physical therapy. You should provide them with case studies or success stories of other people just like them. You could answer their specific concerns or questions that are currently holding them back from coming to see you. You could talk to them about what your costs are and explain how easy it is for them to directly refer to you.

A great Nurture System focuses just as much on addressing the reasons they are currently <u>not</u> booking as it does explaining the reasons they should. Here are three things you might use in your Nurture System:

NURTURE SYSTEM COMPONENT #1: FOLLOW UP PHONE CALLS

Any world-class follow up system includes picking up the phone at regular intervals (after they have seen your ad and made their first contact with you)

The telephone is the primary source of communication in the follow up process and everything else that you will give to the potential patient (after they have requested your free report) is designed to support the work you are doing on the phone. The phone call lets you build a real relationship with the patient and is most likely where they will make the decision to take the next step with you.

With this in mind, at the point of exchanging your free lead magnet (report/PDF) it is critical that you ask for their best telephone number. This allows you to make what I call "check-in", or "progress" calls with them to discuss how they are getting on and to see if/when they are ready to come and see you. It's often the case that a patient who requests the free report will tell you that they want to read your free report first and gives you permission to call back later.

If at this point you make it clear that your true intention is to help her make a good decision and to support her while they do that – however long it takes – it makes for a very positive relationship from the get-go.

This "nurturing" process is vital, because if you try to move them too quickly they will close off from you and never get to truly consider you as an option. If you take the approach that you are supporting them on their journey (as discussed in chapter 3) they will invite you to call them back.

THE PROGRESS CALLS

When you do call them back, what will you speak about? We speak only about things that are important to them. Two questions you might ask them during a follow up conversation are: *"Are you still worried about…?"* Insert whatever their problem is that they first told you about, and *"what other options are you considering?"* The first question continues the conversation about what is concerning them, and it provides a perfect segue that allows you to move the relationship forward with the patient – or end it.

Think about it – there are only two answers to this question. If they are still worrying about whatever their main concern is then you are closer to them saying yes; it opens the door to a conversation about how you can resolve it at your clinic. If they say "no", it means their problems are resolved, and if that is the case, then you wish them well and invite them to call you anytime they need you.

The reality is though, that their problem doesn't go away within a couple of days and they almost always say "yes" (that they are still worrying about it). When this happens, continue to talk to them about how your service can help solve that problem and invite them to take the next step with you.

WHAT OTHER OPTIONS HAVE THEY GOT?

The other question you might ask them is, *"what other options are you considering?"* This forces them to realize that you are likely the only option. At best, they'll say that they are thinking of talking to the doctor or getting some exercises off of the Internet. As soon as they tell you, it is then very easy for you to tell them why your service is the much better choice, especially if they want to achieve the things they told you when you asked the first question.

We've been using these two questions for years now and they really help you get to the heart of the conversation – one you should be having quickly.

How often should you call them back? Well as a general rule you should aim to call them back once per week until they are ready to book or they tell you to stop. Of all of the things you can put in your follow up system, the telephone call is the most powerful, and it is ultimately where the decision to hire you will be made.

"DO YOU LIKE DINOSAURS, HARRY?"

Making these follow up phone calls to the patient is really about finding the one single thing that is going to connect you to them. It is about asking the right questions for however long it takes – until you have found the spark that lights them up and opens the door to an emotive conversation about what they need.

At first, your patients will be a little bit "uneasy" about speaking with you (their mother likely told them not to talk to strangers) and they may find it difficult to tell you what they really want. It's no different to most of us when we first start talking to people we don't know.

For example: if you are sitting next to a stranger on a plane, what can often make the difference between having a great conversation or sitting in complete silence is a baseball hat or soccer jersey!

If the person sitting next to you happens to be wearing your rival team's soccer jersey and you make a comment on it, chances are it will open up a long conversation about your opinions on soccer, eventually leading to other questions like "so where are you from", "where are you going?" Etc. We are often just one question away from a great relationship with someone. The key is to ask questions all the time until you get to that point in the relationship where you are both very comfortable with each other and you can have an open, honest conversation.

Here's an example of what I mean: a couple of years back, one of my most successful Accelerator students and a dear friend of mine, Lois Wolfe from Phoenix, Arizona (of AZ Sports and Physical Therapy), came over to the UK to visit my clinic. Lois came over with her partner, Mark, and one evening we all decided to go out for dinner together in Durham. I picked Lois and Mark up from their hotel. In the back seat of the car was my then 3-year-old son, Harry. Some background on Harry: he is a beautiful, fun, and very friendly little boy. He had once been described as a "social butterfly" by his pre-school teachers, all of whom regularly comment on how easily he gets along with everyone at the school. Normally, he gets on great with most adults, too.

But on this one occasion, when Lois and Mark got into the back seat of the car, he quite literally "closed off from them". As they got in the car and started to talk he immediately curled himself up and looked the other way. This was very unusual for Harry, and despite the fact that he turned away and "cuddled up to himself" (like a frightened little boy watching a scary movie), Lois started to ask Harry one or two questions. She started with the typical "how are you?", "where have you been today?", but Harry wasn't responding.

So Lois changed tracks. She started telling us all a story about how on the day before, she and Mark had been to the National

History Museum in London. She also explained that she had pictures on her phone of the dinosaurs on display down there. All of a sudden there was movement from the car seat Harry was sitting in. We had previously been to the same museum just a couple of weeks before, and when we were there Harry was obsessed with those same dinosaurs. The moment Harry heard the word "dinosaur" he bolted upright in his car seat and turned to look at Lois. Sensing that she had got his attention she asked him this question, "do you like dinosaurs, Harry?" He immediately smiled and nodded his head. The next question she asked was, "do you want to see the pictures of the dinosaurs on my phone?" Harry nodded and quickly took the phone out of her hand to look at the pictures.

From then on, it was a completely different relationship between Harry and Lois – he wouldn't stop asking Lois questions about what her favorite dinosaur was and if she had any videos for him to watch. For the rest of the night they were inseparable and my 3 year returned to the "social butterfly" that we know he is. Moral of the story? Inside every one of your patients is a frightened 3 year old who does not feel comfortable talking to you for whatever reason – at first.

FINDING THE DINOSAUR EQUIVALENT THAT LIGHTS UP YOUR PATIENT

If you haven't grasped the meaning of the story, the ultimate goal of the progress calls is to find the equivalent of the dinosaur in your patient's story – the one thing that lights them up and will open the flood gates for an engaging conversation about their real problems and how you can help them. When you ask the right questions for long enough you eventually strike a chord with the patient, opening up the likelihood of an inseparable relationship much like the one Harry had with Lois that night.

Here's a key point in case you missed it: had Lois stopped asking my son questions after the third time he ignored her, their relationship, and the outcome of the evening, would have been very different. The difference between a social butterfly and a scared little kid was just one question. And likewise, the difference between a patient who is skeptical and one who is ready to book a full plan of care is often just **one question**.

If they are pushing back and resisting then it is a sign you are selling the wrong thing (marketing message) or you're asking the wrong questions. Do not assume that just because they don't engage with you at first it means they are not the right type of patient. It means that you have not found the dinosaur.

If you are ever tempted to think that you keep getting "bad leads", I hope you can hear a guy with a British accent (me) whispering these words in your ear: "find the dinosaur". The right follow up process will get you to that one question and it will completely change the relationship you have with your patients – for the better. Sadly, not long after this evening with Lois she passed away from a very short battle with an illness. RIP Lois and thank you for your support and memories.

NURTURE SYSTEM COMPONENT # 2: EMAIL

If you only add a follow up telephone call (and nothing else) to your Nurture System, then you are already going to be more successful than you are now. But, if you want to give yourself even more chance of success, then layer the communication you are having with your leads by sending them automated emails.

Simply sending two or three emails per week is going to help you stay at the front of the patient's mind between phone calls. These emails are pre-written (using something called an "auto-responder" – I use Infusionsoft), and they contain things like case studies or the success stories of people you have previously helped.

You could write about the top FAQ's of physical therapy (that past patients have asked you), tell people how easy it is to refer to you (explain Direct Access), and give insights into how you can help people get the specific outcomes that they want. Remember, this entire marketing system is built for a perfect patient and the outcome that person wants. At every point we are giving off signals that you know how to achieve the outcomes she wants <u>better than any other option they currently have.</u>

Let me clear something up: despite what some people say, if used correctly email is still one of the most effective forms of media for reaching people (and that is despite its declining open rates). Both you and I are still reading emails that provide us with useful information or are from people we like. Email is not the problem – the junk that people put in the emails, is.

You are not going to be putting junk into your emails, you're only inserting things that are of interest to the patient, i.e. solving the problem or achieving the outcome that they requested information on already.

My clinic's emails are always relevant to the patient. The content is all about them and is constantly showing them how to solve their problem. As a result, I have very little issue with getting my emails read. Sending emails to patients ensures that you are always "top-of-mind", that is, that they are actively thinking about you, so that when you come to make your next "progress" or "check-in" call in 7 days' time, they are more familiar with you. Because they've been thinking about you, it means they are in a better position to ask you better questions and this leads to better outcomes for both of you.

It is not possible to send emails one by one if you are planning on scaling your clinic, so it is best to have them sent automatically. To do this, I use a CRM software called "Infusionsoft" (I've used many and it is by far the best). I'll tell you more about the software and how to get a personal demo at the end of this chapter.

NURTURE SYSTEM COMPONENT #3: DIRECT MAIL

When I first started doing "follow up" my Nurture System consisted of only phone calls and emails. It worked very nicely. But, when I added direct mail to the follow up process, the conversion rate exploded!

Sending people direct mail is important because it not only creates that "omnipresence" feeling that I spoke about in the previous chapter, it also gives my information a better chance of being consumed and understood. We all read and absorb information in different ways, and much of the direct mail that I send is just the same content as I send in the emails, only now it is re-structured and put in a postcard, a letter, or even a "mock" newsletter (just like I do with my attraction ads).

For example: the "mock" or "fake "newsletter is positioned as a monthly clinic newsletter, and this one is, for instance, all about back pain (or whatever their problem is). So, all 4 pages are made up of previously written content that I have used in the emails. The newsletter is something that the patient finds to be very valuable; it allows them to consume what I am saying in a place, and at a time, that is more comfortable and convenient for them. They could read the newsletter at home, in the office, in bed late at night, at the coffee shop, and so on, but wherever it is they do, they are going to be more comfortable doing it, and therefore they'll be more likely to read what I am saying and offering to them.

CASH IS KING, THE 32 PAGE NEWSLETTER

Do not underestimate the power of a newsletter like this. If you are currently sending a newsletter to doctors, it's most likely a complete waste of time; they are unlikely to be read (what doctor do you know with the time to read a newsletter from every physical therapy clinic in town?) However, if you create a newsletter that is dedicated to solving a specific person's problem, then they are very effective and they do get read.

I remember when I first introduced Cash is King, a 32 page monthly newsletter, to the members of my business coaching program. When I first told them about it they didn't really understand it and many couldn't see the value. That was until the day it arrived on their clinic's doorstep…

It is now the most loved and eagerly anticipated aspect of being a member of my coaching program, and because we are able to showcase what our most successful members are doing each month – and how they're doing it – it has become quite addictive for the thousands who read it all over the world.

The monthly publication gets sent out to clinics all over the globe, and it comes with $10,000 worth of marketing ideas arriving on their doorsteps every 30 days. What problem do we solve for our members in the newsletter? How do we ensure that it gets read and people continue to subscribe to it? We make sure that we solve clinic owners' number one problem: where to get proven marketing ideas that successful clinic owners are using. It means our clinic owner members are NEVER STUCK for marketing ideas! This newsletter publication is packed full of ideas and strategies that other business owners, just like you, are using to win more patients and boost profits. So, it is impossible for them not to get value from it, meaning they want to keep getting it.

(If you are wanting to "test-drive" what it is like to be part of the community and receive this monthly newsletter at your clinic, there are details on precisely what's inside my Cash Is King newsletter, here: **www.paulgough.com/wealth-gift.** Sign up for just $1 (cancel anytime) and you'll get a 60-day free trial; you'll also become a member of my Cash Club Program and receive all of the great benefits and privileges that comes with it. Becoming a member of Cash Club is the easiest way to start working with me more closely).

THEY HEAR IT - BUT DON'T ALWAYS UNDERSTAND

For proof of how valuable newsletters can be to you, let me share a true story... I remember a time when I was teaching a clinic from Raleigh, NC, how to do this follow up process. The secretary was using the phone to tell a prospective patient (a lead who had called and requested a free report) that he was able to come down for a free Discovery Visit in order to see how they could help ease his back pain. The secretary had spoken to the gentleman three times already, and each time she had offered the free first visit option – and each time he declined.

A week later they changed the media and they sent him one of these "mock newsletters" I had designed for them. In the newsletter was a big section talking about how to claim a free "Discovery Visit", what the benefits of it were, and how it worked. The guy called up within a day to ask if he could have one of the free Discovery appointments. What he actually said was "why didn't you tell me about this Discovery visit before now?"

The reality is, the secretary did tell him about it, it just wasn't in a place or time that he could process and understand what it meant to him.

Now though, things were different. The newsletter was being read in the comfort of his own home where he could truly relax and process what was being offered to him - what the benefits of coming in actually were. On the phone, he was hearing it, but he wasn't understanding it. **Big difference.** I hope that story sticks with you because, if all you are ever doing is calling them and they keep saying "no" to your offer, most times it is not because they don't want it, it's just more likely they didn't understand what it meant.

Changing the media (much like in the Attraction System) often produces this type of boost in response and conversion, and it is why I recommend that you consider adding some kind of direct mail to your follow up process. Even a simple handwritten note explaining what you have spoken about on the phone, summarizing the offer to come and see you, would make a difference to many people.

It took me just a couple of hours to create these things for my clinic and they're still being used years later. This is another example of how I get so much leverage (more done with less) at my practice.

INTRODUCING "INFUSIONSOFT" – (THE AUTOMATION SOFTWARE THAT I USE TO GROW MY CLINIC WITHOUT HAVING TO BE THERE EVERY DAY)

The obvious next question is, "how do you deliver all of this?"

Well, when I first started doing it I was doing things manually, which made it very time consuming and difficult to scale. After much trial and error, and looking for a software solution to help me automate and organize the whole follow up process in one place, I found a CRM (Customer Relationship Management) software called "Infusionsoft".

Almost every successful business that I was following was using it; I thought that if it was good enough for them, it will be good enough for me! From the moment I found the automation software I knew it was the solution to help me automate and systemize all of this for me. It the heavy lifting out of the process and it is like a member of staff – one that is very cheap and never phones in sick!

Infusionsoft allows you to send pre-written emails, it can keep track of everything that the patient is telling you on the phone, and it allows you to create a dashboard that shows your lead pipeline.

That means I know where all my patients are on their journeys and at which stage they are in with us. It even tells us when a patient is due a call back so that my team never forgets! It tells us how many new leads and inquires we have gotten that day, that week, or month (or year), and it even connects with a direct mail service; this means even my postcards and some of the mailers can be sent automatically.

Infusionsoft is now the powerhouse of everything that we do and it is the primary reason I have been able to grow and scale so quickly. I have no idea where I would be without it. I think I would rather lose my cell-phone than Infusionsoft, as it allows me to automate almost every aspect of my business. It has sky-high email deliverability rates (unlike many cheaper options), and I have nurture and follow up "funnels" (as they are called), for just about every aspect of my business. Whether these are funnels for someone who requested a back pain report, someone who has recently booked an appointment at my clinic and who needs to receive a series of welcome emails and a call right away, or even someone who drops off or cancels, they communicate directly to the patient.

Yes, we even have pre-written funnels and tasks to reactivate and engage these people, and because of Infusionsoft's unrivalled tagging and report capability, most of it gets done automatically and the dashboard is updated in real time. This means my staff know where our patients and leads are at all times. No one is going "missing in action". It is the key to growing sustainably and predictably and something like it, is a vital addition to your marketing dept.

CROWNED "SMALL BUSINESS ICON" BY INFUSIONSOFT

Figuring Infusionsoft out became a bit of an obsession for me. The more I understood it, the more I realized how much more I could do with it. I got so successful with the software, and so much additional revenue was contributed by it, that I was officially acknowledged by the global software company, and in 2016 I was crowned "Small business Icon – Best in Class Lead Nurture and Follow Up". I was chosen for the award ahead of 45,000 global customers for the success I had at my practice using the precise follow up process I have just described to you.

PAUL STYLE INFUSIONSOFT SYSTEMS!

Infusionsoft recognized (and loved the fact) that what I had done was use their software to help people make good decisions about their health whilst simultaneously growing my practice profits. Since the award, I've had physical therapists from all over the world wanting to know how I use it grow my practice. Because of that, Infusionsoft asked me to become a strategic partner in their company. This means that my team and I now work directly with them, and indeed their community of physical therapy clinic owner clientele, to help those clients grow their clinic profits using "Paul Style" Infusionsoft systems.

If you want to see precisely how I use Infusionsoft to grow my clinic, feel free to request a demo by sending an email to paul@paulgough.com with the subject line Alternatively, you can go online and take the free training at **www.paulsinfusionsoft.com** where I'll breakdown the 7 key systems that I use to grow and scale my practice in an in-depth 90 minute free training webinar so you can see how I do it.

I can tell you that having your business automated and powered by systems is truly "liberating"; Infusionsoft CRM and it's incredible capability has been pivotal to my success as well as my ability to scale to four clinics that run without me.

I only recommend things that I have personally used, things that have helped me, and I could not recommend anything as highly to you as I do this software. If you are fed up of trying to do everything in your clinic manually and by yourself, just start with a demo or get in touch to discover what is possible for your clinic. On the demo you'll get to see exactly how my app works and see for yourself what it can do for you.

Try it - I think you will be pleasantly surprised by what it will do for you and how easy it is to get going with "Paul Style" systems that will help you grow.

9

THE CASH VALUE MAXIMIZATION SYSTEM

Now that you've got more calls, more leads, and more patients wanting to pay higher prices, the next thing to do is ensure you maximize the value of each one of them. Most businesses stop short of doing something like this and it is really hurting their profitability, and therefore limiting their chance of growing.

Here's why this system is important to you: there are only three ways to grow a business:

1. To get more customers

2. To increase the amount that the customer spends

3. To increase the frequency of how many times they buy from you

The third and final system in your new marketing machine is called the "**Cash Value Maximization System**", and it is designed to boost all three paths of growth.

Here's how it looks and where it sits in the marketing machine you are creating:

FIG.7

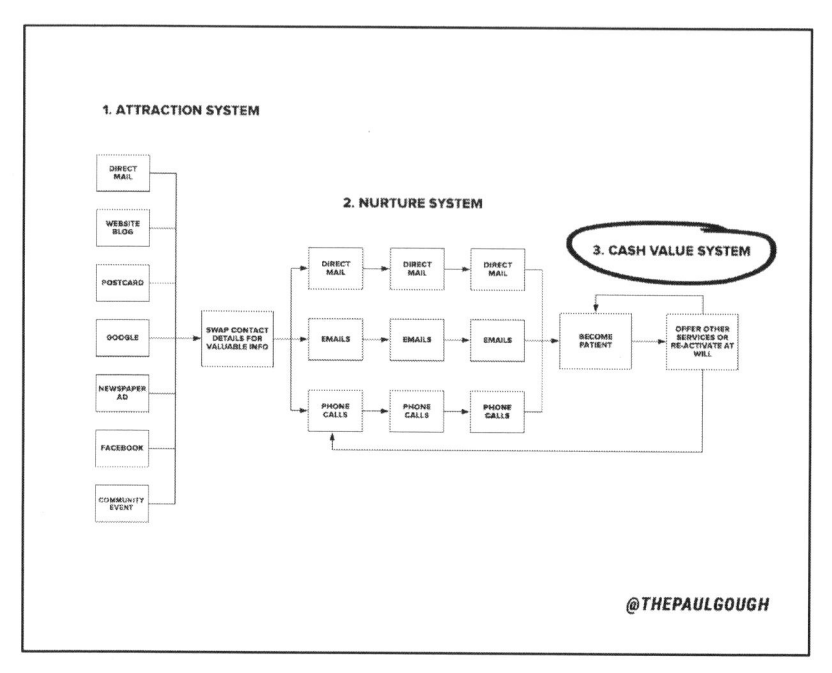

[Diagram showing three systems: 1. Attraction System (Direct Mail, Website Blog, Postcard, Google, Newspaper Ad, Facebook, Community Event) → Swap Contact Details for Valuable Info → 2. Nurture System (Direct Mail, Emails, Phone Calls in three stages) → Become Patient → 3. Cash Value System (circled): Offer Other Services or Re-Activate at Will]

@THEPAULGOUGH

As you can see, it is what happens after your fist two systems have gone to work for you, and without this system you would be leaving a lot of money and impact on the table. Said differently, you've done all of this work to bring the patient through the doors (via your Attraction and Nurture Systems), so it just makes sense to create a system that generates maximum value for both you and the patient.

Here's how we do it at my clinic:

1. **Automate the process of asking for referrals from your current patients**

2. **Automate the "reactivation" process of those past patients who have stopped coming to see you**

3. **Offer those patients something else they need – (something that they're currently buying from someone else)**

To be clear, this is not just about extracting more money from people. It is about adding value to their lives, so much so that they'll be happy to exchange time and money for it.

THE CUSTOMER KNOWS BEST – ASK THEM IF THEY WANT IT

In general, business owners often have a hard time asking people to buy things from them (…and with that mindset, an even harder time paying their own mortgage and monthly bills) even though they know their product or service is valuable.

There's a very simple philosophy that I live by, and it goes like this: "I am <u>not</u> the person to decide if the patient wants to buy or do something – they are!"

The patient, and only the patient, is the one who should be deciding if they want to buy or do anything else with you – or not. <u>My job is to make that decision easier, and it starts with making her aware that something else exists</u>. It is borderline disrespectful of me to keep things that might help her from the patient just because I think she might not want it or might not be able to pay for it. My job as a business owner is to identify WHO the person is I want to help (target market) and then set up a system to offer the things that I believe are suitable for solving their problems. It is then up to the person to decide if they want to buy it.

Many business owners believe that by asking for referrals, sending emails with reminders to come back to the clinic, or offering other products or services, they are somehow "bothering" their patients. But that is not true so long as what you are asking for is ethical and the offer is needed. If my dentist tells me that I need to invest in seeing the hygienist, that if I do it will save me months of discomfort or my teeth falling out, I am not accusing him of selling to me, I am <u>thanking him for it.</u>

I often joke that my business has become a permanent reminder service to my patients – a reminder that they need to come back and sort out whatever health issue they have before they get worse or it gets permanent. **Not** having a Cash Value Maximization System in your business is going to hurt them – and you.

If you are ever struggling with the mind-set or confidence needed to push on in your business, if you struggle doing things like following up with people, raising rates, emailing them, or suggesting that they come back and see you, please never forget that the only purpose of your business is to solve problems. And in our case we solve health problems. Does it get any more important?

Every decision that you make in your business should be guided by the effectiveness of what you're doing when it comes to solving a pre-identified problem for a patient. If you do that, you and your business will do amazingly well, you'll feel great about doing it, and nothing will stop you.

So let's look at each one of these ways to maximize the cash value of your marketing activity in more detail:

CASH VALUE MAXIMIZATION STRATEGY #1: AUTOMATE THE PROCESS OF ASKING FOR REFERRALS FROM CURRENT PATIENTS

Most clinics will wait until the end of the patient's care to ask for referrals from friends or family, but I've found that the best time to do it is within 72 hours of them booking an appointment.

At the beginning of their relationship with you people are excited, they are delighted to have made a decision to hire you, and they are now optimistic about the future. They feel great and they will want to share that excitement with someone they know. Make it easy for them to refer to you by suggesting that they refer people who might need you.

The other thing that people often neglect to consider is that a lot of people would prefer going through the treatment with someone they know. I know my perfect patient, Mary, loves the fact that her friends come for physical therapy at the same time as she does.

It makes it even more comfortable for her and it cements the decision (which improves show up rates and limits cancellations). When birds of a feather who flock together all come for physical therapy at the same time, you're now the thing that they're all taking about in the coffee shop later that day. It only takes one person to overhear and you've got ANOTHER patient…

WHAT TO DO TO AUTOMATE THIS ASKING FOR REFERRALS PROCESS

So, that's why we do it. Here's how we automate the process at my clinic: as soon as someone books an appointment at my clinic our pre-written "welcome to the clinic" e-mail sequence goes out to the patient to, quite literally, "welcome them to the family". Infusionsoft starts to send them their first email within five minutes of booking the appointment and then on day three (after they book), the system sends them another email basically asking them "who do you know that needs our help?".

Of course, we tell them how easy it is to refer people to us – which is standard stuff – but, what we do that really makes the difference in the volume and quality we get, is provide them with "information" to assist in the referral process. We offer them the "free lead magnets" we created in chapter 6.

In the email that gets sent to our brand new patient (on day three after they book) we provide a clickable 'link' to a webpage where they can download all of our free reports. We ask the patient to simply send the email to her friend (who might need us), and then to give the friend instructions about how to fill out the form, which in turn, will help solve the problem the friend has via a report she receives. The email gets sent to the patient's friend, and the friend with the pain clicks on the webpage; she then gets the free lead report that she needed.

They are doing all of this online, so it is 100% automated and the free report of their choice gets sent to them instantly. Can you guess what happens next? That's right, they enter the appropriate Nurture System (the same one that we created in chapter 8 to grow that relationship with your prospective patients).

These potential new patients have indicated that they are interested in getting a solution to a problem we can solve, and what's more, they have given us their contact details. Now we have another "lead" going through our already built Nurture System – the same system is already working for you to bring in people from your external marketing campaigns, and now you are able to use the same system to bring in referrals from past patients. When they enter the system, the automated process of calling, emailing, and sending direct mail to that person, begins.

In my experience these people (referred by patients) need much less nurturing. Their speed of decision in choosing you is much faster. They are already "nearly there". They just needed a little bit of love and a nudge in the right direction to get them over the line and onto your schedule – give it to them from all angles so that they do not procrastinate any longer.

WHY YOU DON'T GET AS MANY REFERRALS AS YOU WOULD LIKE

Giving your patients information to give to their friends' works because it stops your patients from having to become "sales people" for you. This is the biggest mistake most clinics make when asking for referrals – they are asking their patients to do the selling for them.

Chances are patients are telling their friends about you, but they often say the wrong things (they talk about what happens and not the outcome you deliver).

Have you ever stopped to consider what people say about what we do? Picture the coffee shop conversation where a past patient is telling someone about you. The inevitable question is "what's it like", or "what do they do?", and if your patient starts to say things like "well, you have to take your clothes off", "he put his elbow in my back right at the point where it hurt", or "he stretched my leg into a position it has never been in before", they're hardly likely to call, are they? Compound that by how much it costs and they're very unlikely to call no matter how good your past patient's intentions are.

They are saying the wrong things, which is why so many patients who tell you that they will "tell everyone about you" fail to get them to come and see you. They are simply saying the wrong things. That's what this system is designed to stop, therefore significantly increasing the likelihood that the potential patient has an accurate understanding of what you really do. If they have a better understanding about what you do they will make better and more confident decisions to hire you.

So, the solution to more referrals from past patients is to **give them information that they can pass along for you**. The best part is, you already have it (from what you are using in your attraction ads). Now you just need to create a system whereby a patient's friend, colleague, or family member can get it from you.

Think about what this would mean for your clinic: having someone who booked an appointment at your clinic today refer someone else to you within a few days from now. It is as close to "two for one" as you can get, and it really is an explosive way of growing your business, on autopilot, with as much leverage as possible, making it significantly easier for you to grow profitably.

CASH VALUE MAXIMIZATION STRATEGY #2: AUTOMATE THE REACTIVATION OF PAST PATIENTS

Now that you have your Attraction and Nurture Systems in place, you are going to be getting more patients, and therefore, more names in your database.

This is your "customer list", and this list is possibly the greatest asset you will ever own. Managed and looked after properly, your list of past patients who have already spent money with you will give you a bigger return than any house you buy or stock market investment you make.

However, all too often this asset is forgotten or overlooked. And much like any other asset you've got – stocks, shares, property, etc. – it's going to need some attention if you want it to give you a decent return. The key point I want to make from the get-go, here, is that automating the process of bringing these people back to you is very different than waiting for them to come back to you. The difference in many cases could be a $5k profit month or a $10k profit month.

Now, when most clinic owners say they "get a lot of past patients coming back", what they are really saying is that the patients 'finally remembered' that they need to come back in. The clinic is often a passive player in the decision to come back. The clinic is at the mercy of the patient remembering to make the call. That is not a good position to be in, because as you may have noticed, people are not great at remembering to do things like call and make physical therapy appointments.

One thing that I've learned about growing a busy physical therapy clinic is that patients are not great at prioritizing us over other things that they need to do. "I've been meaning to call you for weeks" is the usual line they use. Because of that, I know that if I am relying on people to remember to call me then I could be waiting weeks, months, or even years, and in all that time my profit, and their health, is not going to get better.

What's more, if you ever have dreams of one day selling your practice for a high multiple, and all you are able to say about how you generate patients is that you rely upon "word of mouth", or "past customers", and that there's no repeatable system in place to generate new customers, there's no way anyone would buy your practice for your ideal price. If there is no specific, measureable, repeatable, and scalable process for bringing in new patients or bringing past patients back, then you will never sell your business; you'll always struggle to grow it. Instead of just sitting, hoping, and praying that my past patients are going to come back and see me, I created this system to make it much more likely that it will happen.

MAKE RETURN PATIENTS A PREDICTABLE PROCESS

Here's how we do it at my clinic:

It all starts when the patient is discharged from our care. On the day that she has finished her final treatment session she should be entered into a system that has pre-written emails, includes phone calls, and even has direct mail (in marketing language this is called a "funnel").

It is really very similar to what we do in the Nurture System, only this time we are nurturing them to **come back**.

The message in the emails we send to people who have completed their plan of care will be very different as they already know, like, and trust you. These emails are kick-started by the system when the patient's details are entered into a web form (by the physio or admin) and in my case, Infusionsoft begins to communicate with them asking them to do things like leave us a review or follow us on social media. It even tells them about other products and services that we offer.

STAY IN TOUCH LONG AFTER THEIR PLAN OF CARE IS FINISHED

What we are doing is staying in front of them – staying "top-of-mind" so that they do not forget about us. If you just do that it significantly increases the likelihood they will come back faster. I call this a "lifelong discharge system" because we quite literally stay in touch with them for life. My system sends them emails at set periods of time, for example, at the six and twelve month mark since they were last in.

The emails could run alongside things like postcards, direct mail, and even telephone calls from staff checking in on them. By using something like Infusionsoft I can set "timers" in the system so that on the six month anniversary of the very day they were discharged. (or "graduated from care" as we sometimes call it), they receive an email or postcard (with an offer to come back). The system will also tell someone on my admin team that they need to make a call to this person to discuss coming back in for a review or a check-up. It is all automated, and the message in the emails or postcards is about the offer of a "6 month check-up" or a "12 month review".

At my clinic about three out of ten people respond to these messages sent via email alone, all requesting to come back and see us.

ANOTHER PIPELINE IS BEING CREATED

If you think about how this works, you are essentially creating another pipeline. And that is important, because it is the clinics with the deepest pipelines that are the most successful. If that pipeline is empty and the phone stops ringing, you are in trouble!

Every day that you finish a patient's plan of care and you discharge someone from your clinic, you are filling up this new pipeline. If you have a system for them to enter, it is only a matter of time before people start responding to your emails or phone calls, and because most of it is automated, there is no better return on your time or money.

With the automated reactivation of your past patients taken care of, and now that you have new patients, each of whom is referring more new patients (who will also be in this discharge pipeline soon), it is going to be so much easier for you to grow and scale a very profitable clinic using this method.

Quick tip - if you are a brand new business owner, do not wait. Don't think that you need to have a huge caseload of patients to discharge before building this type of system. If I had my time again I would have done this the moment I had got my very first patient.

CASH VALUE MAXIMIZATION #3: OFFER SOMETHING ELSE OF VALUE

We are not done with making you more profitable yet. There's one other way we can use this system to maximize the profitability of your clinic, to offer the patient something else that they can buy from you. This is actually the easiest way to boost your business profits.

People love to buy things, and so long as you are offering things that solve their problems or will enrich their lives, they'll buy them from you it. Most people are already buying things that they could get from you from other companies. Why not offer it to them yourself at your clinic?

Right now, a large chunk of your database (and future new patients) are online buying things like pillows, orthotics, exercise equipment, clothing, recovery aids, TENS machines, lumbar rolls, etc. Or they are spending money on services like massage, stretching sessions, yoga, or Pilates. Why are they not buying these things from you?

Think about the hassle and time wasted by your patients when they are looking for all of these things. It is significant. I know from personal experience when I have gone online to buy fitness equipment for my home in the past, I'd been overwhelmed by the amount of choices that I had to the point that it actually put me off. I have experienced many situations where I bought things for the gym at home, but in the end they were not what I thought I was buying. This only meant that I then had the hassle of having to send them back and starting over again.

THE SECRET TO MORE PROFIT - KEEP SOLVING PROBLEMS

I've said it many times already: business is about solving problems, and your business will only survive if you solve problems for people.

Do not look at your cash upsell as selling something TO patients. Instead, look at it as something you do FOR people – you're saving them the hassle and frustration that comes with going online: having to decide which items to buy, deciding whether or not it is the right one, whether it'll do the job, having to wait for it to arrive, and so on and so on.

These are the real problems you solve when you offer people other products and services that support their desired outcome. It could even be cheaper for your patients too. If you buy things like pillows or exercise equipment in bulk you will get it at a discount; that means you can then retail it to your patients at a profit and, in most cases, it could still be cost effective for them to buy it from you.

We've been able to add an additional $82.25 to every person (on average) that comes through our doors, simply by offering a very limited number of additional service. These services can include massages, orthopedic pillows, orthotics, and maintenance programs we call "a year of care" (that is, a finite number of sessions people can buy up front at a discount).

This additional $82.25 is very important to me, and not because I take the profit – I actually reinvest it into more marketing; it's important because I am able to fuel the marketing expenditure of my Attraction System with this additional money. And, in doing so I am able to out-spend all of my competition on marketing (which is the ultimate goal and the real secret to sustainable business success). While they are struggling to find the money in their budget for the things that I showed you in chapter 7 (The Attraction System), I am having it paid for from the profit I make on the other problems I am solving for people by using this cash up-sell. That lets me appear in the newspapers every week, be all over Facebook, and get to No.1 on Google AdWords – all because of my additional offerings at the end of the plan of care with me. This gives me real and significant leverage.

This system is a vital cog in your businesses wheel, and I urge you to consider implementing it. If you are a typical "one and done" clinic where people arrive for a couple of sessions and then leave without doing anything else with you, then it is going to be a painful process for you to grow.

HERE'S HOW TO MAKE THE CASH UPSELL PROCESS WORK

When it comes to trying to grow your business by offering something else to the patient, the biggest mistake people make is to wait until the end to offer it to them. That scenario happens because most retail outlets upsell you right at the point of sale and physical therapists want to avoid this trend. In a physical therapy private practice, that is a costly mistake.

From the moment patients book an appointment at my clinic we start to introduce them to the other things that we've got. In the very first email that they get from us (sent to them by Infusionsoft) they are told that we "also offer other things to support them on their journey to great health".

Here's the distinction: in the email telling them about what those other things are, we encourage them to ask us about the products or services and if they think they need any of them. The call to action is "you ask us". With that one email we have reversed the process of selling. In fact, we are not selling – we are offering – and all they have to do is reply to the email and ask us a question or express an interest. When they start to ask you about something, it is a sign that they are considering buying.

No one likes to be sold to - so the answer is to <u>create an environment that they want to buy from</u>. Automation systems really help you to create that type of buying environment, and if you have the right message in the emails that you send to the right people, then those people start to buy more things from you.

It really isn't that difficult, and once again it relies on you having identified the right person to come through the doors in the first place. For obvious reasons, if you are trying to sell the latest super-duper running orthotics to a 70 year old lady, you might find it a struggle. It isn't that people don't want to buy, they just want to buy what is right for what they need, when they need it. This process is made easier with the right front end attraction marketing process in place.

MORE WAYS TO SELL MORE PRODUCTS OR SERVICES

Another way we increase sales of our additional products is to be always bringing it to their attention in the treatment sessions. Sounds simple, but most things that work are. It is the consistent execution of these simple things that most clinics find difficult.

Here's how we do it - during the treatment session you could ask the patient if they like to do things like Pilates, or if they've considered going to a class and what they know about it. You could ask them if they like to get massages, or if they have a regular person they go to and if it's currently convenient for them. Or you could ask if they are happy with their current pillow. Asking your patients quality questions leads to great answers about what they value and their current spending habits.

When we get the answers, we ask for permission to tell them about how we can possibly provide that same service for them. Once they give us permission to do so we go on to tell them all about our option. It doesn't always transpire that people buy things from us immediately after this conversation, but it does start the process, and that is why we need the automated follow up system to help us out.

What we do next is record their interest inside of the customer relationship database (Infusionsoft), and we do this using a simple web form to input some details about what they told us they liked. Essentially, we are building a profile of the patient's wants and needs. The physical therapist needs only to complete a short questionnaire about what the patient said she was interested in (i.e. massage, orthotics, pillows, year of care, etc.) and that information is immediately passed to an appropriate department in my clinic.

In this case it goes to what I call my "follow up team" (the same people talking to the leads we generate from the Attraction System – you could use an admin to get going), so after the treatment is over, they pick up the phone and continue the conversation with the patient about the product or service she has expressed an interest in. We are not actually selling anything. We are **offering** it to people in a way that they want to buy it. Big difference. There's very little push back and the whole process is seamless.

As I said at the start of this chapter, there are only **three ways** to grow a business, and having the customer buy from you more frequently is one of them. Perhaps it is the easiest one.

10

GETTING INTO THE $100K CLUB

So there you have it – your new direct marketing machine made up of three systems all designed to get you more of the right type of patients, make you more profit from doing less, and still get you home by 5pm each night. You've got the **Attraction System**, the **Nurture System**, and the **Cash Value Maximization System** that will power your businesses growth and profitability from now on.

The principles and strategies can be applied to a cash-based, out-of-network, hybrid, or traditional insurance practice wherever you are in the world.

In fact, this method has been so successful that at least one of my Accelerator students has used these same strategies to first grow his traditional insurance clinic in North Carolina, and then start and grow a 100% cash-pay clinic in South Carolina. You can find out more about how he did it, and see his exact marketing strategies on the free webinar that follows this book. **Go here to access it:** www.acceleratorwebinar.com/book

If you are still reading this book it tells me that you are a very serious student of business and that you are committed to the success of your clinic and, you are likely to benefit hugely from the **additional insights I share with you on the free training found at: www.acceleratorwebinar.com/book**

The Accelerator Method has worked for people like you who are from all over the world. Whether you are in America, the UK,

Canada, Australia, New Zealand or Europe – even the Middle East and Dubai – I've got physical therapists using this marketing system to grow their clinics in every economy and in every type of niche. Many have already gotten past **$100k** in additional cash-pay revenue (inside 12 months) since implementing these strategies in their clinic, and it is my wish for you to join that club, ASAP.

I created the Accelerator Method so that you can find the right type of patients who are happy to pay your fees. If the doctors won't answer your call, that's ok – you now have a new strategy that means they are irrelevant in the process of acquiring new patients. If the insurance companies won't pay the fees you deserve, that's ok too – they too are irrelevant because you now have a new strategy to market directly to the cash pay market (who will pay your fees).

Having all three systems in place at your practice helps you get noticed by more of the right people, and best of all, has them understanding the value you bring to their lives and health, long before they even arrive. This makes the conversion to high paying patient much easier; it ultimately ensures more compliance with more buy-in and less push-back when the cash pay or price conversation comes up.

At its heart, the Accelerator Method is about helping people make good decisions about their health. And as it relates to you, it is about positioning you as the stand out provider of physical therapy in a very competitive and overcrowded market place (that is only going to get more saturated as time goes on and more people open up clinics).

This system for marketing your practice is how you will become what I call "beyond dominant" in your town, even if it is packed full of corporate hospital systems and/or cheaper alternatives are freely available everywhere.

Whatever your competition – this is how you will win, regardless.

WHY I WANTED TO SHARE THIS WITH YOU

I wanted to share this system with you for a number of reasons; firstly, to clear up any false beliefs you might have about marketing, to show you that there is a different way, one where you are profitable while simultaneously serving people better. And secondly, to give you the **confidence** that comes with knowing precisely how and why patients choose physical therapists. When you know that it is nothing to do with experience, relationships with doctors, or the size of a clinic or marketing budget – not even the price – it is liberating. This gives you the opportunity to "level up" wherever you are starting from.

I risked my own time and money to figure all of this out, and I've shared with you **proof** that another way does exist for growing your business. You do not need to chase referrals from doctors or feel like you have to remain trapped inside the system with your profits plummeting and stress levels climbing.

Having a marketing system like this also helps you to find more TIME in your business. And time is the greatest gift that any serious business owner can be given. Imagine if you had more of it in your life right now. What would you get done that you currently can't? When you are not doing things repeatedly, and manually, you will find more time in your day to spend on high value activities. Instead of doing trivial $10 per hour work, you are concentrating on high value work that brings in $200, $300, and $500 work per hour. Only when you do enough of that type of high value work does the profit column change for the better.

What is more, you can <u>spend more time with your patients</u>. Because that is what they really want and really value – and that is what world class practitioners want to do also.

Most places treat their patients like "bill-able units", they are always looking for ways to reduce time with patients in an attempt to save money by cutting expenses. This is the fastest road to ruin, and I don't know how any business owner can operate like that – but I know many do.

When your clinic's marketing system is automated, it means you save time; time which can be reinvested back into spending with the patients that are coming to you see you as a result of that marketing system. It is a positive, self-fulfilling cycle. I am speaking from experience when I say that it allows you to develop deeper and more meaningful relationships with those people you are trying to help. While everyone else is trying to rush them in and rush them out (so that they can get the bill to the insurance company), you will have the time to spend with them that no one else can. And they will notice it too.

This ability to find time you currently do not think you have (and being able to give it back to your patients) is a hidden advantage of using the Accelerator system. I know that having this time is what will set you apart from every other physical therapist who is too busy to do the same.

WHAT IS THE ALTERNATIVE?

Take everything that I have taught you throughout this book and use it to build more confidence and trust in your patients' decision to choose physical therapy and hire you. If you do that, you'll be rewarded handsomely for it; you'll have more compliant patients happy to pay higher prices.

After all, what alternative have you got?

The current methods that business owners are using are obviously **not working**. There's a reason we have a debt and stress ridden profession where more and more business owners are taking home less pay than the people they employ.

Finally, I believe it is the people who are willing to give before they get that are successful in this life, and the entire Accelerator system is about giving people what they need and want even before they have to give you anything in return. It is about going back to the fundamentals of how humans build relationships – the Accelerator system is **reciprocity** at its very best.

Yet, despite the simplicity of the message I am sharing with you – that to be successful with your marketing you need to give before you get – I am under no false illusion about how many people will actually do what I am saying. Whenever I speak on stage I tell the audience – no matter how big or how small – that only a small percentage of the people listening to me will actually do what I am suggesting (even though most of them will privately admit that it is what they need). There is a big difference between knowing that something is right – and actually doing it.

Having worked with thousands of physical therapists from all over the world, I can tell you that what separates the world class business owners from the average is **speed to implementation**. The world class business owners, who own businesses that they can be proud of, who have the type of profits that others can only dream about, are the ones who take the same information that others have access to and implement it in their business without any excuses.

They get it done regardless.

Sadly, of the hundreds of thousands of people who read this book in its lifetime, I suspect only a tiny minority will actually do something with the knowledge that is now in their hands.

I sincerely hope that **you** will be one of them, and I look forward to hearing about your results.

A REMINDER OF THE OPPORTUNITY – 15X MORE PATIENTS

Before we end, I want to take you back to the beginning of how this book started, with a look at the opportunity that is staring right at you…

Statistically, the biggest mistake you can make when trying to grow a physical therapy clinic is to try to get referrals from doctors. Studies have proven that there are just not enough of them around for everyone to be successful (see the study by Fritz and Childs, mentioned in chapter 1, and found in your book resource PDF). The only thing you will get by chasing doctors for referrals is tired. And what's more, the next worst thing you can do is to think you can stay profitable when you are trapped inside of a system that is paying you less (insurance reimbursements) even while your expenses are rising.

It doesn't take a NASA genius to work out that if your profit is going down, and expenses are going up, that you cannot win long term. You may get bigger, but you will also be getting less profitable, and *that* is impossible to sustain. Please do not make the same mistake as I did, do not only do something about it when you get a signal from your heart that something is wrong.

The Accelerator Method takes you away from the misery of chasing doctors who won't answer your call and insurance companies who want to pay you less than the cost of running a clinic. It takes you away from fighting over the small 7% of people your competition are all trying to get. Instead, it puts you in front of the MASSIVE group of people who need you – who just need a little "love" from you before they will book.

This system of marketing directly to the public is tried, tested, and proven by not just myself, but the now hundreds of Accelerator Program students who have adopted my "prototype", that is, the new way to market a physical therapy clinic like yours – and they have had stunning success doing so.

You can say that you don't like it, but you can NOT say that it doesn't work. It does. And to my knowledge, the Accelerator Program, and the number of physical therapists using the marketing methods taught in it, is the **largest of its kind anywhere in the world.** I think the reason that so many are using it is because they all recognize that the old-fashioned model of growing a physical therapy business is out of date; it is set up only for the corporate "mill like" clinics to survive (who care about volume not quality), and for those with special relationships with doctors that most of us will never have (nor want to have.)

Now, just in case you forgot what the journey for most clinic owners looks like, here it is again:

FIG.8

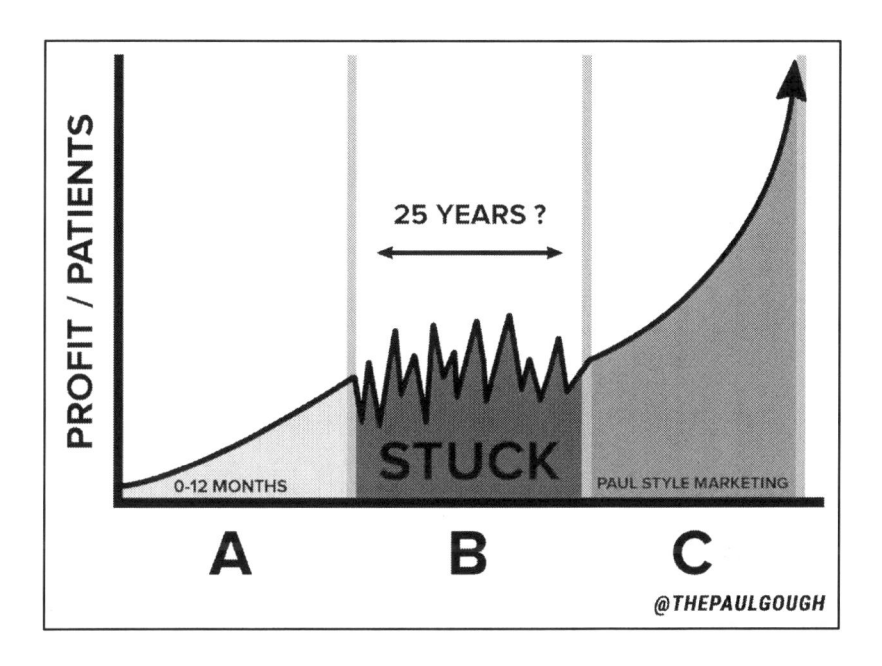

![Figure 8: A graph showing PROFIT/PATIENTS on the y-axis, divided into three zones. Zone A (0-12 MONTHS) shows gradual growth, Zone B shows erratic "STUCK" fluctuations labeled "25 YEARS?", and Zone C (PAUL STYLE MARKETING) shows steep upward growth. @THEPAULGOUGH]

If you are a new business owner reading this book then you are in **Zone A** and you're likely to be working hard or "hustling" to bring in your patients. You are likely to be knocking on the doors of fitness facilities and yoga and pilates studios, you are asking friends and family members for referrals, and you are likely to be using social media to tell everyone in your network that you exist. That is fine, but the problem is that it is not sustainable or scalable, and without a clear marketing strategy to bring in new leads, predictably and reliably, you will get **stuck**!

Those methods might get you started, but they'll also get you stuck! The big mistake is to think that because it worked at first you now just need to do more of it. But that is how you get into **Zone B** – stuck – and like most, you might never come out.

Zone B is where most of the people reading this book are heading. Worst still, you are trapped firmly inside of it already.

It is a painfully frustrating process of doing the same thing over and over – knocking on more doors, posting more on social media, and constantly asking people to refer to you. You watch as your numbers spike and dip, boom and then bust, and you're always feeling like you are working harder with little more to show for the extra effort. There's no certainty in your decisions and everything in your business, from hiring to upgrading your premises, is put on hold because you never feel quite confident or certain that you'll have the patient volume to cover it.

Sadly, most clinic owners stay in Zone B for their entire career. It is a case of "it is not working like we want it to, so let's work harder at it and do more of it to see if that changes anything". It is madness, but that is how so many people are operating right now.

What is needed is not more hard work or more hustle – it is a completely new strategy. You need to enter **Zone C**, where you have a predictable system for acquiring new leads and patients for your practice. The Accelerator Method you have just read about in this book will do that for you.

YOUR OPPORTUNITY TO WORK PERSONALLY WITH PAUL

Just before I leave you, I want to say thank you for giving me your time and attention right until the end of this book. It tells me you are a serious student of business – serious about your business success.

That is exactly the type of person that I love to work with, and because of that I am offering you an invitation to continue to **study with me personally**.

If you have finally decided that you are fed up with waiting for the phone to ring, sick of chasing doctors for referrals, or that you want to avoid being trapped inside of the insurance system and want more cash-pay patients, then there are **two ways we can work together** after this book to ensure you achieve your goals with the least amount of hassle and in record time:

1. FREE ONLINE TRAINING

NEW PATIENT ACCELERATOR: "HOW TO ADD $100,000 IN CASH PAY REVENUE – WITHIN THE NEXT 12 MONTHS"

The Accelerator Webinar is a free and in-depth online training webinar that shows you the exact steps that my most successful *New Patient Accelerator* students have taken to break into my "$100k Cash Club" – the exclusive club for Accelerator students who have added $100k per year or more in cash pay revenue at their clinic since taking the Accelerator Program.

The 90 minute webinar will show you step-by-step (…including example marketing campaigns to look at) how people just like you have moved away from traditional physical therapy marketing that no longer works, to using "Paul Style" marketing that brings in more cash patients and more profits.

You will see iron-clad proof that everything you have just read in the pages of this book really does work and that it really can help you to see more cash patients, make more profit, and still be home by 5pm each night. I will be hosting the free online training personally, and you will be able to submit your questions to me beforehand.

HERE'S WHAT YOU'LL LEARN:

- Step-by-step, the exact marketing system that *Accelerator Program* students have used to **add $100K** to their cash pay revenue
- How one *Accelerator Program* student grew a "traditional" insurance based business – and simultaneously **started a cash-based clinic** (in another state) using the *Accelerator Method* Marketing System
- The exact marketing campaigns that one *Accelerator Program* student uses to charge **$450** per session (…he was charging $175 before Accelerator!)
- How to go from $4000 per month – to **$20,000** per WEEK in cash pay revenue (…and the exact marketing methods an *Accelerator* student used to do this)!

ACCESS THE FREE TRAINING HERE:
www.AcceleratorWebinar.com/book

Choose this option if you want to see precisely how this system is being used by others just like you to bring in more cash and more profit. It is a genuine training (90 minutes), and at the end of the training you will be given an opportunity to enrol in the New Patient Accelerator Program, a 6 week Advanced Master Class where you can work personally with me if you decide it is right for you.

2. ADVANCED MARKETING MASTER CLASS

WORK WITH ME IN THE "6-WEEK NEW PATIENT ACCELERATOR PROGRAM"

New Patient Accelerator is the advanced 6 week Marketing Master Class I designed. It reveals everything you need to know about marketing a successful cash-pay clinic. In this program I share, in much deeper detail, every one of the marketing strategies outlined in this book. I also give you the latest ad templates and examples of marketing campaigns (which are working for me and my clients) so that you can quickly and easily implement these systems into your practice. With this program, you can implement it all <u>with the least amount of hassle, in the fastest possible time frame, and with the most success</u>.

You will have access to me throughout the program; this is the same program that has allowed hundreds of physical therapists to tell insurance companies to "go-to-hell", to say "thanks but no thanks" to chasing referrals from doctors, and to show anyone who ever doubted that they could be successful in business that they were **WRONG**!

It is the exact program that cash pay physical therapists like Kevin Vandi (of Competitive Edge PT, San Jose) used to grow his cash-pay revenue from $4000 per month to $20,000 PER WEEK…that Level 4 PT (of Encinitas, Ca) used to raise their cash pay rates from $175 to $450 per session… it is the same program that Jake Berman (of Naples, FL) took when he had just 4 visits per week on his schedule and was charging just $150 per session, and now, just 18 months later, has his schedule fully packed with 60 visits per week and is charging $225 a session… it is the same program that Trupti Mehta (from D.C) took when she was charging just $160 and had one visit on her books, and who is now charging $250 and seeing 40 visits per week just a year later… and, it is the same program that brand new start-up Next Level PT (of New Jersey) took and within 18 months was making $50,000 per month as a cash pay clinic.

The list of success stories coming in as a result of the New Patient Accelerator Program is growing larger by the day, and if you are finally ready to step-up to the **next level** of business and marketing success, then this is the program that will show you how to do it right.

You will work with me personally for 6 weeks as I give you the "copy and paste" cash-pay marketing campaigns, specific 'how-to' advice on converting cash-pay patients, and provide the tech support you need to implement everything you will learn during our six weeks partnership. I will also connect you with other physical therapists who have already taken the program before you.

Everything you need is delivered to you via a series of instant access videos, PDF scripts, live Q/A calls (with me), and an interactive online community (of hundreds of other Accelerator students), all to ensure that you can put this marketing system into your clinic without any hassle or getting stuck.

ACCESS THE ADVANCED MARKETING MASTER CLASS, HERE:

WWW.PAULSACCELERATOR.COM

If after reading this book you have decided that this type of system is exactly what you have been searching for, and you do not want to wait another minute to have it working at your clinic, then go ahead and enroll in the program now: **www.PaulsAccelerator.com**

The best part is that most of my students see a return on their investment in the program **before they even finish it.**

So, what are you waiting for? Pick which one works best for you and let's get to work!

I'll see you on the webinar or in the advanced master class training program.

To your success,

Paul Gough

P.S If you really are done with chasing referrals from doctors and accepting a pittance from insurance companies; if you know there is a gap in your marketing skills and business strategy; if you really are committed to doing what it takes to achieve the results you desire and deserve; if you are serious about reaching your full potential and breaking through as a successful business owner – then I am committed to helping you to achieve it.

I am the perfect "guide" for you and I want you to know that I am not asking you to do anything with me that I haven't done myself…

I've spent hundreds of thousands of dollars learning everything that I've shared with you in this book. Investing in myself and my business education, is the only reason that I am in a position to write a book like this in the first place. I was not born or blessed with marketing knowledge. I paid to learn it. **Every bit of it.**

Investing in my marketing education is the sole reason I was able to grow my clinic by 413% in 12 months, start and grow four other businesses in two other markets and in two different countries, as well as take care of my family's long-term future by investing in real estate and the stock market.

Despite having invested well over $2 million in real estate and the stock market (all from the profit I've made from my clinics), I would still tell you that there is no greater investment that I have ever made than the investments in my business and marketing education.

A successful, profitable business is the EFFECT. Investing in my marketing education was the CAUSE.

Unsuccessful people live at the effect level of life – they wake up each day waiting for things to happen to them or for them.

Successful people live at the cause level of life – they make things happen for themselves regardless of the environment or their situation.

If you want the appropriate training (the CAUSE) to grow your business successfully (the EFFECT), please contact me through email with any questions you might have – or get going now via the opportunities listed below:

EMAIL ME:
paul@paulgough.com

TO TAKE THE FREE WEBINAR:
www.AcceleratorWebinar.com/book

TO TAKE THE ADVANCED MARKETING MASTER CLASS PROGRAM WITH ME:
www.PaulsAccelerator.com

I am eagerly awaiting your response to my invitation…

ABOUT THE AUTHOR

PAUL GOUGH is a published author (The Healthy Habit), an international speaker, and a former professional soccer physical therapist turned successful clinic owner from the UK.

Paul is the founder of the Paul Gough Physio Rooms – a successful **four location cash pay clinic** he started from a spare room in his home, having had no money and no business or marketing skills. Paul has since scaled his clinic from a zero to $1m + clinic, and what's most impressive is that he's done all that in a country with a completely free "socialist" health care system (that provides physical therapy services for FREE for all residents) as his main competitor.

He is a true small business success story; he is now the owner of five companies, in three different markets, in two different countries - two of those companies have achieved million dollar+ revenues.

Paul is the host of the top rated podcast, "The Physical Therapy Business School Podcast" (available on iTunes, Soundcloud and Stitcher). He is also a "Small Business ICON" WINNER of the Infusionsoft award for best in 'class lead nurture marketing' in 2016, an award which is selected from across all of Infusionsoft's 45,000 strong global customers.

He is widely regarded in America and around the world as a leading authority on *direct to consumer* marketing, and he has a proven track record of helping physical therapists attract cash pay patients, growing their practices, increasing profits, freeing up their time, and radically shifting their entrepreneurial thinking. Every week, 10,000's of physical therapists receive his support/advice online and attend his seminars. His business success coaching programs are almost always full.

BE SURE TO CONNECT WITH PAUL ON SOCIAL MEDIA AND LET HIM KNOW HOW THIS BOOK MADE AN IMPACT ON YOU: @THEPAULGOUGH

GET YOUR FREE WEALTH MARKETING GIFT FROM PAUL, NOW...

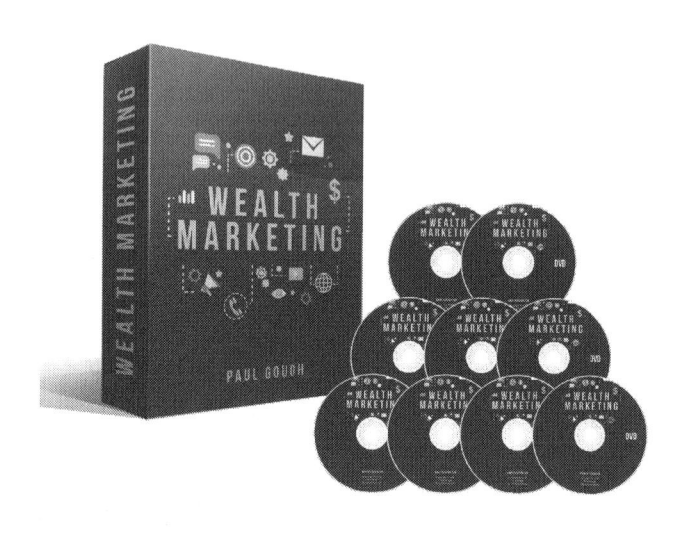

Go to: **www.paulgough.com/wealth-gift**
To get this instant access 9 DVD video program, NOW

Claim your $1,997.00 worth of cash patient generating, higher profit making, wealth marketing DVD program, absolutely FREE!

Including a FREE "Test-Drive" of Paul Gough's Cash Club Membership that sends to your clinic $10,000 worth of marketing ideas every 30 days.

**Claim your copy now, at
www.paulgough.com/wealth-gift**

Made in the USA
Columbia, SC
22 July 2018